"Dr. Ellie has been on my radio show severa͟͟ ͟͟͟, ͟a͟n͟d ͟from her first visit, I intuitively knew she was on to something really important. I immediately took the oral DNA saliva test. Lo and behold, I had a plethora of some undesirable pathogenic bacteria. We've talked to some of the top holistic dentists in the world for over ten years, so I thought I was doing the very best in 'natural' oral care for teeth and gums.

"Dr. Ellie explains in this book what she told me on the radio. I used these strategies to address my problems, and the retest twelve weeks later showed a new state of health, no problem pathogens, and my mouth feels great. Her information is awesome, and so is this book. Looking and seeing and even professional dental examinations have discovered a lessening of gaps between the gums and teeth, after just three months! My teeth have never felt or looked better. The appearance is a more pearly white rather than the much sought after blue-white teeth. Amazing."

—Patrick Timpone, creator and host of One Radio Network

"Great book! You nailed it. A must-read for dental professionals as well as consumers. Over my long career as a dental hygienist and educator, I read and summarized the periodontal research for dentists and hygienists, providing them with the latest scientific findings as well as summaries of classic studies. Over twenty-six years of writing Perio Reports, it was clear to me that a dangerous void existed between scientific evidence and the messages and treatments currently offered in dental practices. Consumers were not benefiting from the science of oral health. They were the victims of outdated traditional messages and treatments rather than true prevention. Consumers follow oral health directions, convinced they will achieve optimal oral health, only to be told at each dental visit that they have more dental disease than before. This is the book consumers and dental professionals need to read to finally understand that dental disease can be prevented with ease, comfort, and for very little money.

"The time has come for dental professionals to realize the old dental paradigm doesn't work. We urgently need to stop blaming patients for their dental disease and shift the focus to protocols that actually achieve optimal oral health."

—Trisha O'Hehir, RDH, cofounder of O'Hehir University, former editorial director of Hygienetown.com, former periodontics columnist for RDH Magazine, and president of Perio Reports Press

"It is well known in the medical field that dental health impacts all the other areas of our health, and yet there don't seem to be any good tools to improve our oral health. Floss more? Brush more? Use this special toothpaste? But very little makes any difference. Until now. When we started bringing Dr. Phillips' information into our clinic and to our patients, the change was startling. People who had dreaded visiting the dentist now came back with glowing reviews. Patients improved their mouths, teeth, and gums so much that the dentist cancelled surgeries. Children *and* adults remineralized their teeth, fixing cavities ... there was so much change that her advice and her programs are a staple in our practice now. You hold in your hands the key to retaining your teeth and oral health for a lifetime, and that will profoundly improve your whole body health. Congratulations!"

—Marlene Merritt, DOM, MS in nutrition and functional medicine, licensed acupuncturist, board-certified bariatric counselor, author, and international speaker

"When we correctly inform people, we give them a choice. This is the power of health education that works. Filled with powerful ideas and easy-to-implement strategies, this book provides the guidance necessary to help anyone gain control over their dental problems. However, its revolutionary contribution lies in empowering you to proactively improve your mouth health and overall well-being. This is a book about hope and a call to stop masking the dangerous underlying problem of a sick mouth by adopting logical, healthy, and common-sense suggestions."

—Dr. Matthew K. Norton, America's holistic doctor, chiropractor, authority on pain, expert in brain science and human performance, international speaker, and author of *Where Does It Hurt?*

"Even the best and most beautiful dental work will deteriorate if a patient is unable to maintain mouth health. A truly healthy mouth will change your dental visits and make them far more enjoyable and motivating. In my office, we have seen Dr. Ellie's strategies improve mouth health, and today, we know so much more about the impact between mouth and general health. This is a book for anyone looking for a new and effective oral care strategy, and I hope many will benefit from the information it offers."

—Sarah Winter, DMD, Sarah Winter Dental, La Jolla, CA

"As certified nutritionists in our 50s, my husband and I believe in living a healthy and balanced life. If we want to be as youthful and vibrant as possible, we need to protect and care for our mind, body, and soul . . . Oral health is such an integral part of this regimen, which is often overlooked. As nutritionists, we *know* that you can't be balanced and healthy without having a healthy mouth. Oral health can be tied to so many negative physical issues, from simple infections to serious issues such as heart and cardiovascular challenges . . . You cannot have a healthy body and bad oral health. The two are intertwined.

"Dr. Ellie is a dental superstar in our opinion. She is light-years ahead of the game when it comes to oral health care. Her program is the best of the best, and her regimen encompasses all areas of preventive dentistry. It is simple and easy to follow. Our personal experience with her program is incredible, and not only are our teeth and gums in great shape, strong, white, and cavity free, but our breath is fresh, clean, and odor free. We wholeheartedly endorse Dr. Ellie's program and can't say enough good about her products, her knowledge, and her dental expertise! She's a rock star! We will endorse and follow her oral health-care program forever!"

—Cheryl Sanders, CN, nutritionist, producer, actress,
stuntwoman, and former WKA World Kickboxing Champion

—Reed Sanders, CSN, certified sports nutritionist,
producer, actor, and extreme sports enthusiast

co-owners, 2Nutritionists.com

"Not every dentist wants to be a leader, become a teacher, or take a stand to improve patient care beyond his or her own office. Dr. Ellie reaches out in her book to empower everyone, from every walk of life, and explain how we can avoid dental problems and improve our oral health. I believe people need this information, and there are few resources that offer such effective and constructive oral care advice. In any arena, it is always personal effort that makes a difference, and the world rarely changes unless we share our passions with each other. This book is a great resource for anyone looking to improve their oral health as it is filled with common sense applications, personal stories, and the latest discoveries in the field of oral science."

—Dr. Ivan Misner, founder and chief visionary
officer of BNI and *New York Times* best-selling author

"My career in dentistry takes me to many countries, helping dental offices through transitions that make their patients healthier. But change is difficult in the dental world, and my work is keeping professionals up to date with evolving ideas and new technologies. Without a doubt, some of the greatest new insights today are about wellness driven dentistry, which Dr. Ellie has explained in this book.

"Like Ellie, I believe it is time for a new approach to improve oral health around the globe. Even small steps, if taken by many, lead to change. As dental professionals, our focus must be the prevention of disease through quality preventive support and long-lasting dentistry. Dr. Ellie's systems are an essential piece of this complex puzzle, and my dental clients are experiencing tremendous success by the implementation of such comprehensive care."

—Cyndee Johnson, RDH, founding principal of scaler2schedule Elite Hygiene, hygienist, educator, entrepreneur, and oral health advisor

"It has been a great pleasure reading the new book by Dr. Ellie Phillips. Dr. Phillips explains the primary causes of oral disease and relates how good oral health is integral to total wellness. By implementing her program, patients can expect better oral health and quite possibly improved general health over their lifetime. I highly recommend this very important book."

—Saul Pressner, DMD, FAGD president, Academy of Biomimetic Dentistry

"Dr. Ellie—Thank you for being a leader that can help us all improve the lives of the people that we care for and treat."

—John C. Comisi, DDS, MAGD, assistant professor, James B. Edwards College of Dental Medicine, Medical University of South Carolina

"Xylitol has been recommended in our practice for a long time, and we always try to make patients excited about oral health. We agree that dentists and their teams should be coaches, advocates, and promoters of oral health. Dr. Ellie has championed the idea of sustainable oral health for years, and this book is a great review of things patients can do to help avoid dental problems. I agree that dentists are an essential part of oral health education and that patients need encouragement to believe that cavities are preventable and why oral health is such a valuable contributor to general body health."

—Christine Landes, DMD, Newtown Dentistry, Newtown, PA, board-certified pediatric dentist, member, International College of Dentists, and ADA council member on dental practice

Ellie Phillips, DDS

MOUTH CARE COMES CLEAN

Breakthrough Strategies to
Stop Cavities and Heal Gum Disease Naturally

RIVER GROVE
BOOKS

This book is intended as a reference volume only, not as a medical manual. The information given here is designed to help you make informed decisions about your health. It is not intended as a substitute for any treatment that may have been prescribed by your doctor. If you suspect that you have a medical problem, you should seek competent medical help. You should not begin a new health regimen without first consulting a medical professional.

Published by River Grove Books
Austin, TX
www.rivergrovebooks.com

Distributed by River Grove Books

Design and composition by Greenleaf Book Group
Cover design by Greenleaf Book Group
Cover images by ©iStockphoto.com/rbv; ©iStockphoto.com/ IvonneW; and ©iStockphoto.com/Antonio-Foto

Publisher's Cataloging-in-Publication data is available.

Print ISBN: 978-1-63299-094-5

eBook ISBN: 978-1-63299-095-2

First Edition

To Margie (1921–2016): My amazing mother, an inspiration, a story-teller, and a lifelong supporter of preventive dental health education. At age forty-five, she was told to have all of her teeth removed, but following my guidance, she ignored this advice and became my first exciting fifty-year success story.

"And let us not grow weary while doing good, for in due season we shall reap if we do not lose heart."

—Galatians 6:9 (NKJV)

Contents

Foreword

Too many Americans suffer the life-changing and debilitating health consequences of diabetes, cardiovascular disease, and rheumatoid arthritis. Medications may help to improve and relieve some of the symptoms caused by these problems, but they rarely address the underlying health concerns. It is my experience that many of these chronic inflammatory conditions can be dramatically improved when digestive health and nutritional balance are addressed. Gum disease and cavities are chronic oral health problems, and as Dr. Ellie explains in this book, toothpastes and rinses can reduce sensitivity or mask bad breath, but the real *reasons* for these problems are frequently ignored and may become more serious conditions over time.

For decades, I have witnessed amazing, drug-free recoveries from many kinds of health issues. These recoveries often appear miraculous when viewed through the lens of traditional medicine, but healing is standard operating procedure for the body when it is provided with adequate support and nutrition. Today, more people have an interest in critically examining their diets, looking for ways to improve their general health, avoid disease, and even reverse health conditions, yet in this search, oral health is often forgotten. Today, we see more clearly than ever before the importance of the mouth as a contributor to the whole-body health puzzle and the fact that dental treatments are not necessarily your only choice.

Of course, a big problem can be sorting through all the information available and deciphering truths from myths. *Mouth Care Comes Clean* helps to do this, discussing science-based research in an easy-to-understand format. Dr. Phillips' career has been in private practice in Europe and the United States, as faculty at the University of Rochester, as a pediatric specialist and clinic director at the Eastman Institute for Oral Health, and as a dentist in senior and special-needs communities. Sometimes we need a wide-angle lens to see more clearly, and it is my experience that some of the best medical advice runs contrary to commonly held beliefs and accepted establishment thinking.

As a nutritional pharmacist, I believe we are moving toward an era where patients, empowered with good advice, should expect to enjoy a lifetime of health and minimal need for medical or dental treatments. This book is a valuable introduction to updated dental concepts, and it should be a must-read for anyone who wants to improve their oral health and learn how to avoid chronic dental disease and the damage it can cause.

—Ben Fuchs, RPH, nutritional pharmacist, founder of
Truth Treatments Skin Care, host of The Bright Side
radio program, speaker, author, and health advocate

Preface

In the past several decades, researchers have discovered so much about mouth health and the hundreds of links between poor oral health and chronic inflammatory conditions that can cripple or debilitate our bodily health. You may think you inherited good or bad teeth, or you may believe your mouth is healthy because you only have a few fillings or a good-looking smile. But the truth is that lack of cavities is not an accurate indicator of mouth health. If you're like countless others, you may have been told that you have no power to change your mouth health, or you may think mouth health depends on flossing or regular cleanings at the dentist. In fact, nothing could be further from the truth.

Mouth health is determined by a delicate biochemical balance that is under our own control each day, for better or worse. Contrary to what you may believe, not all bacteria in your mouth are bad. There are hundreds of good bacteria in a healthy mouth, and the key is to have mouth bacteria in a healthy balance, so they protect your teeth and gums from invasion by harmful, pathogenic ones that can cause plaque, cavities, and gum disease. When certain mouth conditions favor bad bacteria or when certain habits or conditions damage good bacteria, you can start to have dental problems.

It may seem radical for you to view bacteria as beneficial to mouth health or to see your mouth as a living, evolving environment that requires your care and gentle daily maintenance. However, when you digest this new paradigm, it will help you understand why killing bacteria indiscriminately is harmful, why even regular professional cleanings cannot promote long-term or sustainable mouth health, and that unnecessary dental cleanings may, in fact, be potentially harmful.

In the past twenty years, dentists, encouraged by marketing gurus, have promoted the idea of six-month cleanings and marketed this to patients as a way to examine their patients' mouths and find damage to fix. Few patients realize that this damage is caused by harmful mouth bacteria and that fixing cavities and undergoing dental cleanings does not eradicate the disease problem. We know from studies that high levels of health-damaging, gum-disease pathogens are prevalent in the mouths of many young adults and that almost all seniors in the United States are infected. Yet, because gum disease does not necessarily have any symptoms, few people know they have such harmful bacteria in their mouths. Unfortunately, our current system of X-rays and visual examination does not adequately gauge or tell you the true health of your mouth.

The positive side of this news is that mouth damage usually occurs slowly and progressively, and it can be stopped, controlled, and even reversed. To help their patients avoid dental disease and limit the need for treatment, dentists need a better way to measure mouth *health*. Currently, for example, there is no way to take precise measurements that could alert us to negative health changes, so we can know *before* a cavity or gum damage occurs.

Waiting for a cavity to become visible is simply waiting for the bacterial imbalance in an unhealthy mouth to sufficiently damage a tooth to the point at which a cavity will form. Recovery and reversal will always be more difficult after this damage has happened, and it would be a relatively simple process before any visual damage. I always knew there was a better way, and fortunately, with an exposure to Swiss dentistry early in my career, followed by many years of experience and study in a variety of different dental disciplines, I discovered it. My passion for preventing cavities and gum disease was accelerated as more information emerged about the many connections between oral and systemic health. This led me to become a founding member of the American Academy for Oral Systemic Health (AAOSH).

—

In September 2015, I attended an AAOSH meeting and entered their first Oral Systemic Health Challenge. The idea of the challenge was to use the best methods available to gauge mouth health and look for signs of inflammation in the arteries and blood of the attendees. The mouth test was a salivary sample that showed titers of harmful mouth bacteria, sonar testing that illustrated plaque in the carotid arteries, and blood samples that gave clues about systemic or body inflammation. This test was for the dentists, hygienists, and others attending the meeting, health professionals who all value oral health and understand the potentially life-threatening impact of periodontal disease.

The test results were shocking, with most scores averaging only 70 percent out of 100 percent, which was the number allotted for a healthy mouth with no pathogens and no sign of body inflammation or carotid artery plaque. Think about this: These dental professionals who carefully follow the recommendations of the American Dental Association (ADA) were able to achieve only 70 percent out of 100, and most were completely unaware of the many pathogens lurking in their mouths and the plaque in their carotid arteries. Some learned that their carotid artery "age" was as much as twenty-five years older than their chronological age. There was one score—yes, mine—that was virtually perfect at 98 percent.

The reason I mention this is to ask: Why would one score be so different from all the others? I believe that anyone who wanted to do so could use the oral health methods I have used for the past thirty years, and they would develop a similar level of mouth health. I have followed specific strategies designed to nurture a healthy mouth, and I have been tested and found to have a bacterially diverse mouth ecology that has protected my teeth from cavities, my gums from disease, and my body from systemic inflammation and coronary artery plaque. I even wonder if, because my oral care system does not call for flossing, it has protected me from bacteria that could otherwise have entered my blood through gum wounds and potentially deposited in my carotid arteries.

My last dental cleaning was over thirty years ago, and my children have had infrequent cleanings, yet they have all enjoyed terrific mouth health. It is obvious to me that periodic professional cleanings are not essential for mouth health. I would even go so far as to suggest that, for someone with a healthy mouth, professional cleanings can potentially disrupt healthy bacteria and remove a necessary protein layer that is part of the natural mechanism protecting teeth and gums. When your mouth is healthy and disease free, there is no reason for a dentist to aggressively "clean" and disrupt this protective layer, except that it has become an accepted part of modern dentistry's routine protocol.

Please know I am not anti-dentistry. As a dentist, I believe that, if a patient has deposits of infected plaque and calculus, or debris around their teeth, professional cleanings offer them support and will temporarily remove some of the burden caused by this infection. Furthermore, regular cleanings may be a good maintenance system for those who do not care about the health of their mouths and do not want to take responsibility for improving it.

However, it should be obvious that dentistry's protocols are built around a disease model, and this is something I wish to challenge. If you have a healthy mouth and do not need a cleaning, why should we promote regular cleanings that can be costly and may upset or damage your healthy mouth ecology? What if, instead of undergoing a cleaning every six months, you could be examined for any signs of a negative change in your mouth health well before any visible damage? What if you could improve your mouth ecology and avoid cavities and gum disease completely and forever? Well, I believe you can. And in the chapters that follow, I will show and explain the strategies that I use.

The oral care products I recommend are part of a wider strategic plan to promote a healthy mouth ecology that will combat cavities and other problems. My oral care plan can benefit anyone with sensitivity, gum disease, recession, and bad breath when it is combined with strategies for sinus, nasal, and digestive health. The mouth care products I have recommended and used for over thirty years are old-fashioned, over-the-counter rinses and toothpaste that are generally regarded as less effective than the fancy, more expensive, professional-grade, or heavily advertised choices. Later, we will discuss why new stronger or "improved" products may be less effective and why, in some cases, they may even be at the center of your dental problems by causing an imbalance in your mouth's ecology.

Oral care products are only one part of my oral health strategies; however, they are a good starting place. My Complete Mouth Care System features a method of using a specific group of products that have allowed thousands of people to develop, maintain, and sustain amazing oral health for decades. The system evolved as I was working in a busy dental office, questioning patients as I examined their mouth health, because I wanted to know which mouth care products they used.

Over several years, I noticed remarkable patterns and that those using one kind of toothpaste experienced better mouth health. Conversely, I noticed certain products and habits seemed to be causing gum recession and sensitivity, bad breath, or broken teeth. Innumerable patients and clients have used my specific system of care. Often it is necessary to also address their immune system health and daily habits and change their toothbrushing techniques to stimulate circulation in the tissues around their teeth. Only when all these strategies are combined will mouth health improve to its highest level, which will be visible as your teeth become strong and shiny and your mouth feels fresh and comfortable all the time, with gums that do not recede, feel sore, or bleed.

Thousands of people have used my strategies to regain their mouth health and witnessed amazing results. There is no doubt that the most successful were conscientious people who followed my directions carefully. The powerful part of these results is that they introduce a controversial idea: *You can control your own dental future, become empowered, and experience oral health success that will reduce fear, dental expenses, and the need for ongoing dental treatments.* What we do daily, year after year, creates the biggest impact on our general health, and this is the same truth applied to mouth health: Daily care and routines drive health or disease and will determine the outcome for our teeth and gums, for better or worse.

For decades, I've taught my method of mouth care through seminars, workshops, articles, blogs, and podcasts. I've witnessed incredible success stories as cavities vanished and periodontal disease disappeared, sometimes in a matter of weeks! Some of these stories are showcased in my first book, *Kiss Your Dentist Goodbye*, but you'll find many more here. In *Mouth Care Comes Clean*, you will learn more about the connection between your mouth and systemic health, as well as the impact of diet, nutrition, circulation, and your immune system for ultimate mouth health.

Anyone who has read my first book knows I am respectful of my profession and was a founding member of AAOSH. I passionately believe that oral health is an essential component of good general health. I was an active board member of AAOSH when I published *Kiss Your Dentist Goodbye*, which was my effort to interpret dental science so that patients could be empowered to know which habits and products could help them prevent cavities and gum disease and even reverse those problems. At the time of publishing, the book was viewed with skepticism by peers who had never learned that teeth can remineralize or heal themselves. Today, however, most dentists and hygienists talk about remineralization, and many recommend my system of care and have witnessed cavities reverse and dramatic improvements occur in their patients' mouths.

I wrote *this* book to share the most recent science about mouth health and empower you with some additional knowledge that can transform and elevate your dental health to a state where you may no longer need any dental treatments or even cleanings. As we discovered in the AAOSH Oral Systemic Health Challenge, dental and medical professionals using the well-promoted routines that focus on brushing, flossing, and dental cleanings could not achieve ultimate oral health, and many of their results showed signs of systemic inflammation, which is a serious problem for general health. This suggests that our standard recommendations for oral care are not sufficiently comprehensive or effective.

It is an unfortunate fact that 95 percent of Americans, even those who meticulously follow this traditional dental protocol recommended by the ADA, end up with cavities, fillings, implants, lost teeth, and gum damage or disease, which generate ever-increasing dental expenses for these people, particularly older adults. New advances in oral microbiology have changed our understanding of oral health.

My belief is that successful mouth care requires a three-part strategy that will:

1. Balance your mouth biology to create a healthy oral ecosystem
2. Promote maximum mineralization of your teeth
3. Support your digestive health to maximize the absorption of nutrients and minerals that support saliva and nourish your immune system, which aids tissue healing and regeneration

When you have a healthy mouth ecosystem, it can support as many as nine hundred different kinds of bacteria, and so your fight for oral health is actually not to eliminate bacteria but to control a very few—probably around twenty—that multiply in specific conditions to cause oral damage and disease. This means that most of the bacteria in your mouth are harmless and even beneficial. Therefore, instead of using therapies that aim to strip or eradicate mouth bacteria and its associated biofilm, I will teach you how to cultivate a sustainable, healthy mouth and enjoy the benefits of this ecosystem as it works to protect your teeth, gums, and even your general health.

This new approach can help you avoid many of the costly dental restorative treatments and minimize much of the accompanying fear, pain, and inconvenience. This does not mean you stop having dental visits. However, it does mean they should be different, with a focus on ways to determine and learn if your mouth is becoming healthier. Your personal dental health is within your control. Regardless of your genetics or past experiences, you can take charge of your mouth health, and you can start today—even if you already have fillings, have been told that you are a hopeless case, or think your teeth are too crowded or beyond help.

I firmly believe that anyone can improve their oral health, but it does require effort and good daily habits. However, the benefits from following my Complete Mouth Care System are vast: A truly healthy mouth requires minimal maintenance. You may need an occasional cleaning, but if you follow this program carefully, you can avoid the continuum of ongoing filling repairs that turn into root canals, crowns, bridges, or implants. Please know I am not suggesting you avoid going to your dentist. Instead, I encourage you to find an ethical and caring one who is happy to help monitor your mouth health, give you accurate reviews to build your confidence, and let you know that your efforts are taking you in a good direction that will allow you to enjoy *and maintain* a healthy mouth for the rest of your life.

In the pages ahead, I will share the oral care strategies that I believe can help you develop and sustain a healthier mouth. I also will point out the dangers of using certain oral care products and the habits that can disrupt healthy bacteria and upset the mouth ecology that we need to protect our teeth and gums at every age. The sooner you start, the sooner you will stop any dental problems and deterioration in your mouth. I look forward to showing you how to achieve low-maintenance dental health with my easy-to-follow plan. If you're ready, let's begin!

Acknowledgments

This book is only possible because I was gifted such an unusual career in dentistry. My father believed women should have professional equality, a revolutionary concept in the United Kingdom in the 1960s. My parents gave me the opportunity to study science at the prestigious Cheltenham Ladies' College, knowing such an exceptional education would prepare me for dental school. It did, and it was also where I met my lifelong friend and fearless supporter, Helen from Northumberland. My dental teachers included John Featherstone and Edwina Kidd, two revered dental-science icons, even today. Swiss dentistry introduced me to the importance of lifestyle and diet, something that proved invaluable.

My unsuspecting children became a living testimony to my journey as a dentist, suffering the poor outcomes of various techniques I had been taught and believed would make teeth healthier. I am grateful my oldest daughters do not hate me for giving them tooth-damaging fluoride supplements, and my daughter with sealants understands that, at the time, I did not know better. My son reached adulthood with great teeth, but his experimentation with different oral care products weakened his teeth and resulted in fracture. My youngest daughter was possibly the most fortunate as we left her teeth alone, with nothing more than good daily care. Even her wisdom teeth erupted naturally, which had no effect on her perfect smile, even though she was warned this would cause crowding. I'm thankful that my family taught me so much and allowed me to be a busy mother and a passionate advocate for dental health.

My kids have always cheered me on, and so have many dental friends, especially Dr. Randy Freeman, who taught me the art of perfect crowns, and Dr. Saul Pressner, who introduced me to exceptional filling techniques at the Academy of Biomimetic Dentistry. When my family needed help to repair fluoride-damaged incisors and fractured teeth, I was grateful to know two gifted cosmetic dentists, Dr. Corky Willhite of Metairie, Louisiana and Dr. Michael Woolwine of Austin, Texas. Our family continues to revere the skills of these great dentists, who were able to perfectly restore the disfigurement caused by fluorosis and fracture.

Innumerable patients remain in contact with me and their successes and appreciation are great encouragement. I cannot thank them enough for all the questions, emails, and many conversations over the years. These interactions helped me understand the acute dental struggles that worry people and how oral health can become a life-changing concern.

As I entered the business world by making xylitol products, I had great support from many good friends, including biology expert Dr. Michael Rudy and xylitol expert Dr. John Peldyak, who encouraged me on my educational mission to teach about xylitol and introduce this amazing product to the United States.

I appreciate the support of Dr. Marlene Merritt, who is a highly respected Alzheimer's consultant in Austin, Texas and who constantly introduces my system to other health professionals at her seminars around the country. As we enter an era of lifestyle medicine and dentistry, I find myself constantly talking to people who are extremely interested in learning more about oral health as we chat in airports, at concerts, in checkout lines, in the bank, and even during Uber rides! People find the idea fascinating, and when they achieve success, they share their stories far and wide with family and friends. This is how we can change the world through a grassroots effort and how true health prevention may finally reach the people it needs to reach.

Finally, I have to thank the Greenleaf Book Group publishing team: Nathan True, Carrie Jones, Dan Pederson, Diana Ceres, and Nichole Kraft for their amazing expertise and for helping me complete this project. At times, the task seemed daunting, but they offered organized enthusiasm, reminding me why this message is so important and why this book needed to be written.

Many thanks to you all!
Ellie

CHAPTER I

The Evolution of Dentistry

Do nothing, say nothing, and be nothing,
and you'll never be criticized.

—Elbert Hubbard

In the early 1900s, there were many physicians and dentists who believed that diet and nutrition were the keys to oral and general health and that teeth had an impact on whole-body health. From this conviction grew the idea that it was vital to rid the mouth of infected teeth, and this concept is in close alignment with our understanding today. Unfortunately, this observation of how mouth health affects bodily health was often abused and used as a scapegoat by physicians when they were searching to explain or find a reason for an intangible health problem.

The result was that health-care providers recommended many unnecessary extractions in a vain effort to solve unrelated medical problems or improve general health. This scenario led to many perfectly good or savable teeth being sacrificed. The term *focus of infection* was used to describe the suspicious dental source that appeared to be related to these health problems, and in this era, there was no understanding about bacteria or any way to X-ray teeth. Gradually, the focus of infection became a rejected and despised idea, as it was seen as a form of medical quackery. This explains why filling damaged teeth was suddenly embraced as a more professional, lucrative, and glamorous kind of dentistry.

Ironically, at this exact period, a silver-mercury-amalgam filling material emerged in America just as extractions began to become less desirable. The pendulum quickly swung in this new direction, and dentists were soon in the business of saving every damaged tooth possible with this new filling material from France. As this transition occurred, medicine and dentistry rapidly split into separated disciplines and continued to divide further as medical and dental specialties were formed. These subspecialties created the false impression that parts of the body, and definitely teeth, were somehow disconnected from the rest of the body and in no way an influence on whole-body health.

THE AMERICAN DENTAL ASSOCIATION

Looking back, it appears obvious why super-specialized doctors and dentists became myopic as they focused their attention on small and specific parts of the human anatomy, as if those were separated from the rest of the body. These changes took dentistry far away from the science of medicine, and in the mid-twentieth century, a group of powerful restoration-focused dentists became galvanized into a new organization called the American Dental Association (ADA).

The ADA taught and encouraged its members to save as many decay-damaged teeth as possible, using their newly available silver amalgam material. The dental-restoration era blossomed, and there was a surge in the numbers of companies and laboratories creating all kinds of new filling materials, crowns, bridges, and precision attachments that could camouflage tooth damage and fix teeth to avoid extractions. The dental-material companies flourished and supported the ADA in its growth, as everyone worked to repair severely broken, damaged, and infected teeth. Dentists became ever more skillful in their ability to help patients restore and retain their teeth—even dead ones—patching them up and masking infection, so the tooth could survive for years and sometimes for a patient's lifetime.

We understand the excitement this generated in dental circles and how happy patients were to save their teeth, especially when the restored teeth were shades brighter than their old natural ones. In hindsight, of course, we know that most of these fabricated smiles looked shiny and white at first glance, but under the surface, things were different: Rotting dental problems often existed around the tooth roots, and almost all these mouths remained infected. We can only wonder about the impact these good-looking restorations had on the general health of these patients, who sported teeth covered by fake crowns and roots stuffed full of plastics and pastes.

Besides the potential damage caused by the various toxic materials that have been used in dentistry over the past hundred years, even more damage may have been caused by harmful bacteria that were ignored in these patients' mouths. Mouth acidity is a powerful risk factor that promotes unhealthy mouth bacteria. This was also the era when fast food, soda, snacking, and processed foods became popular, and these things probably compounded the perfect-storm conditions for poor mouth health. Underlying dental infections continued to be ignored, and as long as teeth looked good, everyone was happy. The sad part of this story is that cavity- and gum disease-causing bacteria in these patients' mouths were unwittingly transferred to other people in their circle of family or friends, which may be why so many families in the United States today have experienced massive dental problems and a heavy burden of dental expenses.

A NEW FOCUS

Dentistry continued to focus on skills to beautify teeth and methods to repair dental damage throughout the 1980s, and this became reflected in the way dentists were being trained. When I was a student in the 1960s, our conversations at dental school were usually about how to stop or prevent cavities and gum disease. Two decades later, popular topics were about techniques or materials that could turn ugly teeth into a beautiful smile and which innovative products and evolving materials could help speed or simplify this process.

In the 1980s, TV shows promoted dental makeovers, sponsored by companies with a vested interest in igniting a hunger for this exciting form of cosmetic dentistry. Complete mouth rehabilitation was a moneymaker for everyone—product companies, dental associations, and dentists. Even when the makeovers were excruciatingly expensive, the public was mesmerized by the idea of younger-looking teeth and bigger, whiter smiles.

Financing and marketing companies were next to enter the dental arena, with many incentives for a patient to act now and pay later. This was the instant dentistry people wanted—crowns, veneers, and a mouth of the whitest possible teeth, even if they were porcelain, completely fake and often unnecessary. Fueled by demand, cosmetic dentistry exploded, totally ignoring any of the underlying diseases that caused the original disfigurement or dental problems. Dentistry paid little or no attention to the imbalance in patients' mouths, often fueled by acidity, poor diet, or legions of harmful bacteria. These underlying problems were forgotten or ignored in the excitement of a "smile presentation." This presentation was a glamorous ceremony that often occurred in a dental office after the final crowns were fitted, frequently with a semiprofessional photo session for the patient, as he or she smiled wide to show this incredible new makeover. As long as the teeth looked good, dentist and patient were ecstatic.

There was a similar emphasis on perfect-looking teeth for children. Concern shifted away from the mundane education of parents about nutrition, transmissible bacteria, and the real cause of cavities to the new goals of rebuilding teeth with crowns, often at great expense and sadly putting children's lives at risk under general anesthesia. You can fix and fill every tooth in someone's head, but harmful bacteria will remain and continue attacking more teeth to cause additional problems in the future. Teeth become damaged in babies and adults when unhealthy mouth bacteria exist within an infected mouth ecology. Without an effective whole-body health strategy, these harmful bacteria will continue to live in the mouth even after pretty crowns have fixed the damage, and they will eventually go on to cause more cavities in other teeth. There may be arguments for and against the fixing of baby teeth, but there should be no excuse for allowing this awful disease to live in a child's mouth when the antidote is simple, easy, and effective.

DENTISTRY TODAY

The problem with traditional "dental prevention" is that it embraces aggressive mechanical techniques and products that are designed to strip or kill mouth bacteria. Most antiseptic rinses and antibiotics do not discriminate between good and bad bacteria and generally end up killing both. Hygienist cleanings will mechanically remove debris and temporarily lighten the disease burden in an unhealthy mouth, but sustainable mouth health is only achieved with a kinder, gentler, and more natural approach that supports healthy bacteria and encourages them to thrive. If we nurture the hundreds of good bacteria in our mouth, they will create and build a healthy ecology that can protect our teeth and gums from physical, chemical, and thermal damage and from disease.

You may be shocked that the ADA's recommendation for six-month professional cleanings and daily flossing has never been shown to change mouth health from a bacterial standpoint. My belief is that inappropriate treatments and products can do more harm than good to your mouth either by masking the underlying problems or by causing a bacterial disturbance—or *dysbiosis*—to a healthy mouth ecology. Hygienists are trained in protocols designed to reduce infection, but this does nothing to improve a mouth's underlying ecology. This is why I believe dentistry needs a new approach to help interested patients prevent and reverse gum disease and cavities. Most dentists think it is pure luck if you enjoy a lifetime of oral health without fillings and gum disease. This is why deteriorating oral health is frequently accepted as normal and is seen as an acceptable and regular part of aging, since dentists see this kind of infection and damage in 95 percent of US adults over age sixty-five. By the time you finish this book, I hope you will believe that sustainable oral health is not only achievable but is vital to minimize your risk for chronic general health problems.

Dental Marketing

Ultimate oral health is so precious that it must be protected, which is why I believe it is necessary to question some accepted dental treatments and find out if they upset a healthy mouth and tip it out of balance. Obviously, the idea of less treatment is unlikely to be readily promoted in dental offices, so it is important for you to have a good understanding of what you may wish to have done, or avoid having done, when you are in the dentist's chair. Many dental-marketing companies have enthusiastic partnerships with dental offices. Marketers have a traditional understanding of mouth health, compounded by a goal of helping dentists sell more of the products and services they believe are a benefit to you and a source of income for the dental offices. Recall visits are always an exciting priority for marketers. To them, these visits are the perfect way to boost your health and the dentist's income as a win-win for everyone. These marketing companies encourage a keen focus on the efficiency of scheduling recall visits, which is why you receive so many text messages to remind you about the necessity for your recall visit.

The difficulty is that science does not support six-month professional cleanings as a benefit for a healthy mouth. Frequent cleanings could weaken teeth, thin your enamel, and cause sensitivity by the removal of a vital protein layer, which may leave your mouth more vulnerable to damage and cavity bacteria. A study published in the *Journal of Dental Research* in 2013, "Patient Stratification for Preventive Care in Dentistry," was carried out by researchers at the University of Michigan Medical School of Dentistry and showed no difference in tooth-loss rates over sixteen years with differing intervals between cleanings for low-risk patients. This is no surprise when you understand that cleanings do not improve the ecosystem of the mouth or change the composition of the mouth's resident bacteria.

The study did show that more frequent cleanings helped patients who were at high risk, and this makes sense, as the burden of infection was temporarily lightened—but it was not taken away. A news release by the ADA was published on June 10, 2013, in light of this study, and recommended that, to maintain optimal oral health, regular dental visits should be at intervals determined by a dentist and that their frequency should be tailored and personalized to accommodate the current oral-health status and health history of each patient.

When we feel we are a target of aggressive marketing, it is easy to incorrectly assume that dentists are motivated by money, but we know even ethical and caring dentists can become victims of money-centered sales systems. This is why it's important to be empowered with some dental science yourself and to have enough facts to decide which treatments to accept, which to refuse, and which ones to talk over with a trusted advisor before agreeing to treatment or prepaying for work to be done.

The Treatment Ladder

Dentists have gained a well-deserved reputation for being some of the nicest and most trusted professionals in the world, but most dentists know there have been dramatic changes to the way students are being trained recently and in the way modern dentistry operates. Dentists often graduate with a heavy burden of student debt on their shoulders and enter the workplace without experience and with no time to question their dental training. Compounding matters, the dental business has become more challenging today, and it is harder for an independent dental office to grow in the crowded dental-services marketplace.

This explains why corporate dental franchises have become dominant and a major employer of new dental graduates. Businesspeople usually lead these corporate dental chains, and this has changed the landscape of dentistry in various ways. Certainly, these corporate offices are convenient, but, just like franchised food, there are unfortunate side effects that the average consumer does not always recognize.

For example, it may surprise you to know that many corporate offices begin each morning in a "huddle." Because costs are attached to every type of dental procedure, it is often part of the process for these businesses to coordinate with dental insurance plans and maximize their income and the profitability generated by specific treatments. The office team is taught strategies to guide you "up the ladder" of treatment options, often pushing you toward whitening, a bite guard, or an upsell to cosmetic straightening, crowns, or veneers. As you hear the suggestions from various staff members, you may begin to believe your teeth really need to be whiter or straighter. Staff may even try to persuade you to get treatment before a special offer expires. If you feel a sense of urgency in the pitch, my advice is to beware!

Sometimes, these tactics are targeted toward you when your treatment plan was never finalized. The team's goal is to persuade you to complete treatment, hopefully that will benefit your teeth. In some situations, a front manager will start a conversation to uncover ideas that could maximize acceptance and learn about your dreams or fears, such as an upcoming wedding or an event that could be used for motivation by the treatment coordinator.

In the worst situations, these sales pitches are choreographed ahead of time, and words are specifically chosen to drive acceptance. This effort is obviously acceptable if the end goal is to improve your oral health through honest education, but it is totally unacceptable if it is used to generate treatment, or if less expensive options exist, or if you can reverse these problems simply by improving your home care.

Fillings: Never-Ending Maintenance

Traditional dental care that works to fix cavities and clean teeth has no ability to control mouth bacteria with these treatments. The infection that causes the tooth and gum damage will remain after these treatments, and it will continue to attack your teeth even after all the cavities have been filled. Dentists can restore your teeth to function, but they have no power to change an infected mouth. This is why most fillings become reinfected in about ten years and need constant replacement and repairs that usually become larger and more complicated every time.

Cavities rarely occur on a single tooth, because the bacteria that cause them are everywhere in the mouth and attack all the teeth at the same time. This means that four teeth in mirror positions in each jaw will usually develop cavities within a short time period or even simultaneously. With correct care, a cavity can be stopped and reversed, heal naturally, and never need a filling.

The methods that I teach to reverse a cavity will adjust the health of your entire mouth and improve the health of all your teeth, everywhere. Deciding to fill a cavity that can be reversed has financial ramifications far greater than most people would expect or calculate. For example, similar teeth are usually damaged simultaneously in other places in the mouth. A small filling will need ongoing repairs, which weaken the tooth structure at each replacement and can potentially lead to the need for a root canal or crown.

One small filling that costs only a few hundred dollars and that may have been "covered" by insurance can create escalating expenses that propel the cost into thousands of dollars as the filling needs constant repair and the tooth structure deteriorates over time. Remember, dental disease is preventable, and cavities in the early stages are completely reversible. Think about how much money, time, and aggravation an effective strategy could save you over your lifetime if you decided to reverse the first small filling.

The anatomical locations where cavities occur are places on a tooth surface that have vulnerability to bacterial attack. The most susceptible areas of the most vulnerable teeth will succumb first, and the sequential decay pattern in the mouth is usually predictable, dictated by the relative susceptibilities of different tooth surfaces. This means an experienced dentist will know where to expect a cavity first, next, and so on. This is also why similar teeth usually have cavities at the same time and in similar locations on their surfaces.

Imagine a filling is placed in a child's molar at age six, and this filling needs to be replaced in ten years. Let's assume the cost of one filling is $200 for the first treatment. Now multiply this cost by four molars and potentially six or more repair cycles during the child's lifetime. This cost is now thousands of dollars for a total of over twenty-eight fillings for these four molars. Now imagine three or four teeth on each side need a filling. This can quickly translate into great expense and more than a hundred treatments. In the days when amalgam was the usual filling material, these ongoing repairs created a huge toxic burden for these patients, and may have provoked more dire and negative health consequences in later life.

Some people are proud to have replaced their old mercury fillings with white ones, and although this may be an option, the first concern should be to evaluate the mouth's overall health and, if necessary, take all the steps outlined in this book to improve it. White fillings have been called "plaque magnets," and I believe almost all dental materials, be they silver or white, are dangers to our health, since there is mercury in amalgam (silver) fillings and the plastic compound BPA in white plastic fillings and in sealants. Ceramic material is unyielding, and the constant biting contact against a hard crown can cause fractures of opposing natural teeth. Before having any new fillings or old fillings repaired or replaced, I suggest you take a few months to improve your mouth health with my suggestions, so your new fillings will have an improved chance of survival in a healthier mouth environment.

Periodontal Treatment

The focus of traditional dentistry has been to fix cavities and other tooth damage for almost a century. Only recently has it become common for dentists to take a serious look and consider their patients' gum health. The American Academy of Periodontology's guidelines for gum disease stress that periodontal health should be "achieved in the least invasive and most cost-effective manner." They say this can be accomplished through nonsurgical periodontal treatment, but few patients realize that the majority of treatments done by periodontists are quite invasive, since they often involve deep scaling and root planing, laser procedures, antibiotics, or therapies with trays of peroxide, which may be worn in the mouth for years and possibly forever.

There is a depressing saying: "Once in the periodontist's chair, always in the periodontist's chair." The problem and the reason for this is that most periodontal specialists have never witnessed mouth health that has improved or periodontal damage that has reversed, so they believe you need frequent and ongoing professional treatments and cleanings for the rest of your life. Frequently, the blame for this lack of resolution is placed on the patient, fate, genetics, or inadequate flossing.

The most important message in this book is that fillings, cleanings, flossing, and even extracting teeth do nothing to change mouth bacteria or improve the mouth's bacterial ecology. Harmful bacteria may be moved by mechanical techniques, but these bacteria cannot be eliminated from saliva by these methods. This is why cleanings can only reduce debris and temporarily reduce the numbers of harmful bacteria. After the cleaning, harmful bacteria will quickly relocate from saliva and continue their attack on your teeth or gums. *Peri-implantitis* is a fancy name for an infection around dental implants. Dental implants are the artificial replacements for teeth that have been extracted, often following attachment loss and periodontal disease. Peri-implantitis is basically a resurgence of the same damaging bacteria that caused the original gum destruction and bone loss; essentially, the bacteria have regrouped and sprung back into action to attack the gum and bone around the implant.

Before you commit to any cleanings, extractions, or dental treatment, I urge you to learn as much as possible about mouth health and adopt a plan that will create a healthy mouth ecology. You may be surprised that I advise you to do this *before* any dental work, even before a filling, crown, or implant. The important thing is to understand that you want your new dental work to immediately enjoy the benefits of your healthy mouth and to have a better chance of lifelong survival and less chance of becoming infected or damaged.

DO YOU NEED CLEANINGS?

As we have discussed, periodic dental cleanings cannot make your teeth stronger, cannot change bacteria, and cannot permanently make your mouth healthier. If you have an infected mouth, cleanings will reduce soft and calcified debris and harmful bacteria, which is a help, but a cleaning has no power to stop the underlying imbalance or change an unhealthy mouth into a healthy one. In fact, if we measure the number of disease bacteria in the mouth before a cleaning, we may see their numbers decline on the day of the cleaning but rise a few days after it. To understand why this occurs, consider harmful bacteria to be like weeds in a garden. Weeds can reseed and even multiply as they are shaken and scattered. We will explore in more detail the accurate description of *plaque* in chapter 3. Right now, we need to understand that plaque becomes a problem in the mouth when harmful bacteria multiply and expand within a thin protective mesh that naturally covers the surfaces of our teeth and gums. This protective mesh is an oral *biofilm*, and if you are ever able to notice this layer as a visible plaque on your teeth, this is telling you that the biofilm in your mouth has become infected. There is no healthy "quick fix" to change the health of oral biofilm, but it can be slowly and progressively adjusted to become healthy, and this will happen as you employ effective strategies regularly, using good home care and habits over several weeks. It's always better to improve your mouth health slowly, and I suggest that you work for a few months to develop a really healthy biofilm *before* having a cleaning. At first, you may not stop the need for your next cleaning, but as your mouth health improves, the need for these dental cleanings should gradually reduce, and your mouth will begin to remain healthy for longer intervals between cleaning appointments.

Remember that most dentists, especially younger ones, have been educated and conditioned in dental school to believe dental problems will automatically spin out of control if you do not come to six-month dental appointments. Dental professionals believe these visits are *the* way to preserve your teeth, and this has been their motivation to keep you coming back so regularly. As you surprise your dental professionals, my hope is that you will make believers out of them.

Few dentists are willing to discuss how many of their patients have deteriorating teeth, even their regular six-monthers. Most dentists witness disease and damage day in and day out and have never considered if cleanings could be a negative contributor.

Progressive dental deterioration is frustrating for patients and for caring dental professionals, who may agonize over the fact that they are unable to control cavities and gum disease. The truth is a dentist has no power over the disease in your mouth any more than a doctor can control your bodily health. Doctors and dentists can monitor and evaluate your health, but it is your daily habits that in most cases determine the actual outcome over time. Like general health, oral health is influenced by a variety of things called risk factors. These are the habits, products, and specific conditions that promote an unhealthy mouth environment. This is why the strategies I recommend target a combination of problems, yet they work together in harmony to overcome disease while providing overarching support for the kind of ecosystem that leads you to mouth health.

Many people have been conditioned since childhood to believe they must brush and floss and have regular dental cleanings to "clean" and thus save their teeth. Some people are even fearful that a cavity will develop *because* they delay a cleaning. Parents take children for cleanings, thinking it is the loving and dutiful thing to do, unaware there may be no benefits for a child with a healthy mouth. Worse yet, I believe in some cases these cleanings may be detrimental.

People should not be scared and emotionally stressed about the arbitrary six-month cleaning periods. If you have been told that you have an unhealthy mouth and need cleanings, then the first thing you should consider is a new way to care for your mouth. Until you find a solution that gives you mouth health, regular cleanings will be helpful, but they should not be viewed as a long-term solution. Cleanings may delay the demise of your teeth and gums, but you can have cleanings every month and never achieve ultimate oral health or even an improvement to your mouth health.

If you want better mouth health, you must learn effective *daily* care and habits that support healthy bacteria, protect your teeth from damage, and nurture mouth health. A healthy mouth feels clean and comfortable, it has no plaque, no calculus buildup, no recession, and no sign of cavities, bleeding gums, or periodontal problems. A healthy mouth does not need a cleaning, which could potentially scratch or thin the enamel; more importantly, a cleaning may remove the thin layer of healthy protective proteins and the good bacteria that are the foundation of a healthy mouth ecosystem.

Your mouth certainly should be professionally evaluated at regular intervals by your dentist, and at these appointments, I encourage patients to inquire if their mouth *needs* a "cleaning," even if your insurance is prepared to pay for it. Anyone who is told that they do need a cleaning is someone who has not yet achieved a balanced mouth ecosystem. Of course, many people decide to place the responsibility of mouth health into the hands of their dentist, and these people will always need to rely on regular cleanings as an established maintenance system that can keep their oral health in an acceptable state. Just remember we know that about 95 percent of US adults, even those who have regular cleanings, experience a steady deterioration in their dental health and need more fillings and repairs, crowns, root canals, extractions, implants, and even dentures in their final decades of life.

If your mouth is unhealthy, a cleaning will remove diseased plaque from around your teeth and gums for a time, and this will temporarily help to limit the amount of damage and inflammation in your gums. The more infected your mouth, the more often you will need cleanings. Cleanings can indeed help to slow down the destruction that infected plaque creates, and your dentist's recommendations about the frequency of your cleanings should be gauged to try to help keep your mouth health at a clinically "acceptable" level. The hope of your dentist is that he or she can slow your disease and reduce dental damage to extend the life of your tooth by several decades. A truthful dentist will admit that eventually you will likely need periodontal surgery, bone grafting, extractions, implants, and potentially even dentures. If you have been told that your teeth need cleaning, this is an indication that your home care strategies are not sufficiently effective. Perhaps certain risk factors are creating difficulties for your teeth and gums. Just as pills from a doctor can make a sick person feel better, they do not *make* the person healthier. Regular cleanings may make your mouth feel and look better and delay the demise of your teeth, but cleanings by themselves do not make an unhealthy mouth healthier.

People with a healthy mouth should not need a cleaning. Some people with healthy mouths will get extra cleanings, because they are confused and think that the more they have, the healthier their teeth will be. This idea is upside down, and such frequent cleanings can erode and weaken the hardest part of tooth enamel and make teeth more sensitive, more easily stained, and more likely to crack and become infected.

Stripping healthy biofilm from teeth during a cleaning can put your mouth at an increased risk of picking up a new infection. Years ago, some studies showed how a cleaning allowed cavity bacteria to infect mouths that had been cleaned, because it had stripped away the naturally protective biofilm layer. Strange as it may seem, healthy bacteria have mechanisms to defend our teeth from intruder bacteria. There may also be some degree of danger from bacteria that become splattered and airborne in dental offices, sprayed into the air as teeth are drilled. In 2016, sixty-eight children in Anaheim, California, were hospitalized and contracted severe medical complications after picking up an infection from bacteria in the dental water lines at a dental office.

NEW TECHNIQUES AND EQUIPMENT

For almost a hundred years, dentistry has been a reactive, or late-warning, system, with its primary task to find tooth and gum damage *after* it has occurred. Dentists and hygienists wait and search for decay or gum disease, but few patients are ever warned of impending problems. Thankfully, we should soon have equipment that can give us measurements of harmful bacteria in our mouth and show us the strength of tooth enamel. These tests would be able to alert us to a change in our oral health so that we would know if there are a growing number of bad bacteria, a gradual weakening of enamel, or some impending gum and dental problems long before they could be classified as gum disease or a cavity.

Receiving a dental health warning would allow patients to go home and use strategies to improve their mouth health and avoid the need for treatment. This information would be far more useful than probing or X-rays that are used in dental offices today. Imagine being told your teeth are getting stronger and the imminent cavity had gone away. This approach is a different paradigm that I hope dentistry will embrace, as it begins to focus more on health. Routine monitoring will show progress and allow dentists to watch cavities as they reverse and see the teeth heal and get stronger. How much more exciting is this paradigm than the current system where we wait for a cavity to grow large enough to be found on X-ray or be deep enough to need a filling?

At present, such tests are not generally available, and patients will be instrumental in requesting this kind of care. I believe that patients will quickly grasp the benefit of being alerted to negative changes before there is damage that constitutes a danger or a weakness or before a cavity requires a filling.

SUSTAINABLE ORAL HEALTH

As you can see, dentistry has evolved over the past hundred years. Some of the advancements, such as the new ways to test the health of your teeth and mouth, can be of great benefit to you. What if you could minimize dental costs and simultaneously reduce the pain, frustration, guilt, and annoyance that often accompany dentistry's traditional approach? Would you feel confident about extending the intervals between your appointments if you believed it would help you achieve a better level of oral health?

American dentistry of the twenty-first century has become a massive industry composed of huge corporations that sell dental equipment and materials, marketing gurus that coach dental businesses, and associations that control dental training, manage insurance company alliances, and lobby in Washington. Most people love and trust their personal dental team with very good reason, but there is a lot of science and new preventive thinking that is not currently taught in dental school.

Changing a powerful business and professional conglomerate is not going to be easy, and change-makers are often unpopular. But change will occur, and it often seems to happen organically when a truthful idea is carefully planted and given time to grow. My hope is that this book will help you modify your personal thoughts about oral health and slowly change your dental experiences as you improve your oral health for life.

CHAPTER 2

The Effect of Dental Issues on Your Health

*It's not enough to do your best; you must know
what to do, and then do your best.*

—W. Edwards Deming

In this chapter, we are going to discuss how dental problems can affect your overall health. For example, poor gum health can ignite an area of inflammation and stimulate a reaction that can spread to affect other areas of the body and lead to serious chronic inflammatory health conditions. Poor oral health and the chronic body inflammation it creates can increase your risk for heart attack, stroke, diabetes, dementia, certain forms of cancer, Alzheimer's, and preterm birth.

A healthy mouth will reduce the chance of inflammation in your gum tissues, which may prevent many of these distant problems that can ravage your health. If you have been diagnosed (or if you have a family history of) chronic inflammatory disease, especially diabetes or cardiovascular problems, please consider your mouth health and how it may be affecting your general health. You may want to have a saliva test to check the levels of mouth bacteria we know are implicated in a variety of chronic health problems. An ultrasonic scan can show plaque deposits in your carotid arteries, and a blood test can indicate the level of inflammation in your body. When these tests are combined, they can give a useful warning or indication of the presence of chronic inflammation, which could have a serious impact on your life now or in the future.

Many of my dental and medical friends were shocked when they took the aforementioned tests and discovered a number of unsuspected problems. These medical professionals took immediate action, because they realized the implications of plaque in their coronary arteries and the consequences of body inflammation. They understood the serious nature of these risks and how life-threatening medical events are often triggered by inflammation that can be initiated by certain kinds of harmful mouth bacteria.

TRANSMISSION OF DISEASE

Dentists have known for a long time that dental disease is a transmissible bacterial infection and that this transfer occurs from person to person, from tooth to tooth, and from teeth to toothbrushes, even after a single toothbrush use. It's impossible to prevent the sharing and spread of mouth bacteria as they float in the saliva that moistens your mouth. Within the mouth, saliva is in contact with other nearby anatomical areas, such as the nose, pharynx, throat, and ears. You may brush your teeth thinking that you are cleaning away plaque from your mouth, but your newly brushed teeth will almost instantly become repopulated with the same oral bacteria that will immediately drop out of saliva or spread from confluent areas—places in contact with the mouth, but where a toothbrush cannot go.

The bacteria in your mouth are invisible, and they invisibly transfer in droplets of saliva. Mouth bacteria can generally be classified as healthy or unhealthy, which means you will share your personal variety of bacteria with the family or friends who live around you, and these bacteria will be potentially useful and protective or harmful and aggressive. For a hundred years, dentistry has focused on fixing teeth, and most people have believed that tooth damage is the result of a problem called plaque.

Dentists are skilled at repairing teeth and are well trained to restore the look of your smile and a tooth's biting function. The hygienists' role for decades has been to clean away the debris of infected plaque from around your gums and polish your teeth to make them shine. Dental professionals may try to help you by suggesting toothpastes or rinses known or proven to kill bacteria and strip plaque from the mouth, sometimes for up to twenty-four hours. These routinely accepted approaches focus on ridding the mouth of germs and plaque, but in the long term, killing or scraping away mouth bacteria indiscriminately will not help you develop a healthier mouth. Dental disease is a unique infection as it involves an intricate film called biofilm that covers all the mouth, teeth, and gum surfaces. The health of biofilm is maintained or improved by adjusting your mouth conditions to achieve balance in the mouth's chemistry, physics, and biology. The kind of bacteria in your mouth are changed very slowly over time, which is why it is impossible for a dentist to make your mouth healthier at infrequent dental visits or by killing all the bacteria in your mouth. *You* alone have the power to control this complex situation and develop great oral health using good daily tooth care and habits that promote dental healing and mouth health. The good news is that I am going to teach you effective strategies that create healthy conditions in your mouth that will not only strengthen your teeth but will also help you to develop a healthier mouth biology, or ecosystem. These same strategies will protect your gums while your mouth health improves, but our ultimate goal is that your own healthy mouth ecosystem, supported by your own healthy saliva and your own immune system, will eventually be your primary defense against cavities and gum disease.

MY FIGHT WITH ACNE

The science of skin health has also changed over the past fifty years. My personal experience was the agony of following ineffective skin care advice as a teen. I had acne and a face covered in blemishes, and the teachers at my English boarding school told me that my skin was dirty and the solution was a good daily cleaning with soap and a scrubbing brush. I made painful efforts to scrub my skin and cure my problem, but as you can imagine, all the washing and scrubbing did not solve anything. In fact, the more I scrubbed, the worse my acne became. In addition, my skin felt tight, itchy, sore, and painful, and it was still covered in blemishes!

After years on this demoralizing merry-go-round, I was introduced to a simple three-part routine for delicate skin: a gentle liquid to clean my skin, another to balance my skin's chemistry, and a final lotion that was protective and soothing. I don't remember exactly, but I'd say it took less than two weeks for my problems to miraculously vanish and for my skin to feel comfortable and look fresh and healthy. How was it possible to improve years of bad skin without brushing or scrubbing? It was a long time before I could answer this question and only after I understood that, in the world of health, the goal should never be to strip or sterilize but to create the conditions that support health. Today, we know that skin must be hydrated, nourished, at an optimal level of acidity (pH), and protected by a film of healthy skin microbes and proteins.

I am forever grateful to the cosmetic Clinique consultant in the 1960s who in one afternoon helped me solve my skin problems and changed my approach to skin health for life. This kind lady with her simple outreach was the person who motivated me to think differently and help many dental patients escape a similar "brush and floss" agony and find a more effective solution for mouth health. The correct dental advice combined with specific oral care products can create the environment for quick and almost miraculous changes in mouth health, even after years of damage and disease. For thirty years, my friend and nutritional pharmacist Ben Fuchs has formulated products for skin care that respect the body's biochemistry, and like him, I am convinced that our body is designed divinely to heal and renew itself on a moment-to-moment basis when it is given correct care and adequate nutritional support.

GUM DISEASE AND BODILY HEALTH

The links that connect our mouth and body health show us that oral health is far more precious than sweet breath or a shiny grin. We now know, for example, that bacteria from the mouth can travel in the blood to locations elsewhere in the body. In your bloodstream, these bacteria can cause damage to vital organs like the heart, heart valves, or surgically replaced joints, like a knee or hip. Oral bacteria can also create inflammation and ignite an inflammatory response that can ripple around the body, triggering problems that are not always recognized as coming from bacteria hidden under the gums. The bacteria that cause some of the most serious medical problems lurk in the gums, and from this location, they contribute to dangerous and even life-threatening health problems. There are about eleven kinds of these bacteria known to be involved in chronic inflammatory conditions, and they are collectively known as periodontal pathogens.

Periodontal disease is the name given to a gum infection that is triggered by specific periodontal bacteria. These health-threatening bacteria can multiply easily when they find a secluded place in your mouth where the oxygen supply is limited. Periodontal problems are usually painless, and there are rarely any symptoms or signs of swelling or bleeding. Hidden in a tiny space under the gums, these invisible periodontal pathogens can attack the gums and also cause widespread body inflammation; some bacteria may even gain entry and flow in the blood to other parts of the body. Most patients will be completely unaware of any problems, but their internal body defenses notice these attacks and will try to stop them. Periodontal pathogens are very resistant to the body's internal defense system and also to most traditional dental therapies used against them. This creates a situation where there is an ongoing fight between these pathogens and your immune system, and this fight can continue for years, generated by pathogens in gum pockets around teeth. There is no sign of damage at first, but the longer the situation remains unresolved, the greater the body's response. This is why the unusual inflammatory reaction from gum disease can lead to bone loss around teeth, the loss of gum attachment, and the eventual loosening of teeth. This inflammation can also be magnified if its effects travel around your body. The reaction becomes slowly exaggerated and amplified as it spreads, sometimes triggering debilitating or life-threatening health conditions like rheumatoid arthritis, cardiovascular disease, or dementia.

Most of us will have a few periodontal pathogens floating in our mouth, drifting in our salivary liquids. They should be in very small numbers in a healthy mouth—their presence is normal and will cause no harm. Periodontal bacteria only become problematic if they find a place to multiply. This is when their numbers will increase in saliva. For this to occur, the bacteria need to locate a dark space with limited oxygen. If they find such a space, they will seize the opportunity to lodge and flourish. This is why periodontal pathogens often become trapped under the gum between the tooth and the tooth socket, inside a space called a *periodontal pocket*. Measuring the levels of periodontal pathogens in your saliva is a good way to know if you may have a periodontal pocket somewhere in your mouth.

Because these bacteria are problematic only on occasion, they are classified under the umbrella name of *opportunistic* bacteria. In other words, they need a specific opportunity to multiply and cause harm. The extent of gum damage can be roughly illustrated by calculating the surface area in a mouth with multiple dental pockets. Healthy teeth should have no pockets, but if you had a pocket depth of 5 millimeters on one side of your teeth, this would be an open wound with a total length that is the distance around the mouth (approximately 762 millimeters). If your pockets were 5 millimeters deep, this would create a surface area of 3,810 square millimeters (which is equivalent to the surface of a 6-inch square). No doctor would ignore a festering 6-inch skin wound for years, yet many adults live with this undiagnosed problem in their gums, sometimes for decades.

When you have a mouth teeming with bad bacteria, no amount of brushing or flossing will get rid of them. In fact, I suggest that flossing may actually aggravate the problem and potentially create more pocket opportunities, open up wounds, and even push bacteria into the blood, which could increase the risk for an inflammatory response. I know this is the opposite of our generally accepted dental mantra, but this is why I do not think it is safe for anyone with an unhealthy mouth to floss. It's important to note that flossing was born in an era before periodontal pathogens were understood or could be measured.

My belief is that flossing can actually increase someone's risk for general health conditions that are influenced by poor oral health. These are all medical conditions, such as heart attack, stroke, high blood pressure, rheumatoid arthritis, insulin instability for diabetics, infertility-treatment failure, and preterm birth. This is why, if you want to floss, I suggest you first ensure your mouth is as healthy as possible and maybe take a salivary test to know your levels of opportunistic mouth pathogens before you begin. In addition, gum-disease pathogens have been implicated in the predisposition to certain kinds of cancer, digestive problems, and even dementia and Alzheimer's. In the past, people believed that there was a connection between early tooth loss and dementia, and in 2017, a systematic review of studies on this subject by N. C. Foley and others confirmed an association between poor oral health and dementia more definitively.

Scientists at the Harvard School of Public Health showed recently that gum disease may be linked to pancreatic cancer. Pancreatic cancer affects more than thirty-three thousand Americans each year and kills more than thirty thousand, making it the fourth leading cause of death from cancer. The Harvard studies showed that men with gum disease were 63 percent more likely to develop pancreatic cancer than those without gum disease. In a group of nonsmoking men, those with gum disease were twice as likely as those with healthy gums to develop pancreatic cancer.

Chronic or recurrent sinus infections, middle-ear infections, respiratory problems, and even acid reflux may also be associated with poor oral health. Improving your mouth health will often help relieve the symptoms and recurrence of sinus and acid reflux problems, which is understandable when we think about how the ecosystem of the mouth contacts the ecosystem of these areas. New information is constantly being gathered about the associations between oral health and general health, so please stay informed and check my website, www.DrEllie.com, for the latest studies about these oral-systemic links.

CONDITIONS ASSOCIATED WITH DENTAL AND GUM DISEASE

- Cardiovascular disease
- Stroke and high blood pressure
- Preterm birth
- Cancer
- Diabetes
- Arthritis
- Dementia and Alzheimer's
- Joint replacement failure or slow healing
- Infertility-treatment failure
- Chronic sinusitis
- Middle-ear infections in childhood
- Acid reflux symptoms
- Respiratory infection and pneumonia
- Crohn's disease and irritable bowel syndrome

Heart Disease and Other Damage Caused by Oral Bacteria

Heart disease is largely preventable, but nearly one million Americans have a heart attack each year, with an increasing number occurring among younger people. Almost all doctors and cardiologists today view cardiac disease as the result of inflammatory damage. The main focus of preventive cardiac care is to eliminate or reduce every potential source of inflammation, yet oral health is often forgotten, or flossing is recommended, which I believe may put patients in harm's way. This is why it seems essential for anyone who is at risk for heart disease or stroke to consider my strategies to improve their mouth health and take a salivary test to find out the levels of periodontal pathogens that may be lurking in their mouths.

Salivary testing identifies the number of periodontal pathogens in your saliva and scores the measured levels of each pathogen. A high titer suggests that specific bacteria are multiplying fiercely, which indicates a problem likely exists in the gums, and this could trigger inflammation elsewhere in the body. There are a variety of suggestions about how to control opportunistic pathogens, and of course, the popular ones are antibiotics, strong antiseptics, multiple and deeper cleanings, or killing the bacteria with trays full of peroxide (which are worn at night) for the rest of your life. Later, you will read about my strategy to control these pathogens by nurturing the healthy bacteria in your mouth. If you discover high concentrations of periodontal pathogens in your mouth, you must make a decision which approach to use and take action to stop gum problems before they ruin your general health.

Please realize that, if you accept the normally recommended products and treatments, your end goal will be to kill and mechanically remove biofilm from every surface in your mouth. In this situation, you will need to continue killing or removing biofilm and pathogens, possibly forever. The reason you will never gain control is that this treatment damages healthy bacteria at the same time. An alternative approach is to be considerate of healthy mouth bacteria and use strategies that change the ecology more slowly while nurturing useful and good bacteria. This takes time and relies on commitment by you and help from your immune system. By using a nurturing strategy, however, you should see improvements in your periodontal health within six months and be able to reach a stable state of mouth health within a few years, hopefully something you will be able to enjoy for the rest of your life.

Dentists know that, during a dental cleaning, or even while flossing, it is possible for mouth bacteria to be pushed through the gum and enter the bloodstream. Your immune system usually destroys invading bacteria, but certain strains may bypass these defenses. If you have a compromised immune system, you are at even greater risk.

Mouth bacteria can grow on damaged heart valves and cause a potentially lethal condition called *endocarditis*. Mouth bacteria have also been isolated from other places in the body: around the joints of artificial knees or hip replacements, in heart muscle, in the brain, and in the placentas of pregnant women. Mouth bacteria have even caused the fatal septicemia of an unborn baby and have been isolated from plaque deposits in coronary arteries following a heart attack. Everyone should take mouth health seriously, especially if you are contemplating a new hip or knee replacement, or you are going to have heart surgery, become pregnant, or are being treated for risk of stroke or high blood pressure.

In the past, scientists have had difficulty cultivating certain kinds of bacteria, and this made it difficult to know if periodontal pathogens caused coronary artery disease. It now appears that *Porphyromonas gingivalis* (*P. gingivalis*) is the primary bacteria that erodes gum tissues and enters the bloodstream to travel around the body. *P. gingivalis* have been found in joint tissues, heart plaque, and placenta. *P. gingivalis* has most recently been linked to a higher risk for esophageal squamous cell carcinoma, a type of pharyngeal cancer.

In 2012, UK researchers found that *Streptococcus gordonii* (*S. gordonii*) can masquerade as a human protein and blood-clotting factor called fibrinogen, which allowed these bacteria to attract platelets and cause clumping inside blood vessels. Microbiologists at the University of Rochester found aggressive strains of *Streptococcus mutans* (*S. mutans*), the bacteria of *dental caries*, or tooth decay, had invaded heart muscle, showing how bacteria from the mouth can wreak various kinds of havoc elsewhere in the body.

Gum Disease and Preterm Birth

There appears to be a strong relationship between gum disease and preterm births, and *P. gingivalis* has been found in the amniotic fluid and placenta in cases where babies were born prematurely. Marjorie K. Jeffcoat has investigated this very probable connection between poor oral health during pregnancy and the earlier delivery of babies, which can put babies at risk for many medical conditions, including respiratory problems, long-term disabilities, imperfect organ development, vision impairment, hearing loss, mental developmental disorders, and even death. Because mouth health is generally measured by visual examination—without any bacterial testing—there have been contradictory results in these research studies, some supporting and some negating this link. Dr. Jeffcoat's large prospective study in 2001, published in *The Journal of the American Dental Association*, showed a significant association between preterm birth and periodontal disease when oral health was measured between the twenty-first and twenty-fourth weeks of pregnancy.

In a study published in *The Lancet* in 2008, researchers found less connection between dental care and preterm birth, yet other studies by Nestor J. Lopez in 2002 indicate that, when a mother has a dental cleaning during pregnancy, it could lower her risk of preterm birth. These studies seem to conflict with each other and with studies led by Bryan

S. Michalowicz, published in *The New England Journal of Medicine* in 2006, which showed dental cleanings did not reduce the risk of preterm birth once the woman became pregnant. All the studies used traditional metrics for measuring disease and the old dental paradigm that assumes a dental cleaning, scaling, and root planing is beneficial. What we do know is that, if a mother enters pregnancy with good oral health, she will lower her chance for a premature birth by up to 84 percent and possibly more.

A study in 2014 by Dr. Kjersti Aagaard at Baylor Medical College in Texas has also shown that a mother's mouth health will influence a newborn's digestive microbiome *before* birth. The bacteria found in the placenta after birth matched the bacterial community found in the mother's mouth, and this demonstrates how bacteria can travel from the mouth via the blood and reach the placenta. From the placenta, microbes can reach the baby either by crossing into the baby's blood within the placenta or by passing into amniotic fluid, which is swallowed by the baby. The team also found that specific bacterial species were more common and others less common among women who had given birth prematurely—before thirty-seven weeks of pregnancy. Dr. Aagaard speculates that, if oral bacteria reach the placenta through the blood, then it is possible that bacteria from diseased and bleeding gums could colonize the placenta, potentially triggering premature birth.

This is why it seems essential for a pregnant mother to maintain healthy teeth and gums during pregnancy. Pregnancy is a time when the mouth becomes acidic, and this can easily upset a previously healthy mouth ecosystem. No one should ever accept bleeding gums as normal, especially during pregnancy. If this happens to you, I recommend you take a salivary test to find out your levels of periodontal pathogens so that you can take action and support your immune system to reestablish mouth health. You can learn more about periodontal pathogen testing at www.DrEllie.com.

SUPPORT FROM A DENTIST

Dr. Ron Phillips practiced dentistry for forty-three years, and during those years in private practice, he, like most dentists, believed that dental problems were caused by plaque on teeth. Forty years ago, plaque was viewed as *the* enemy, and this was why plaque needed to be destroyed. Dr. Ron will admit that his passion as a caring dentist was to kill and destroy plaque and mouth bacteria, because he believed the only good bacteria were dead ones. He did not have a hygienist, so he cleaned all of his patients' teeth over those years, which made him extremely conscious of his patients' mouth health. Despite a fastidious patient-training program and the fact that most of his patients were compliant with his brushing and flossing instructions, the vast number of them continued to have cavities, sensitivity, recession, enamel erosion or abrasion, gum infection and disease, and sometimes tooth or root fracture. In fact, Dr. Ron found these problems so common he eventually decided this state of poor oral health could be regarded as normal, especially as people age.

Dr. Ron and I met at a conference on heart disease. We were discussing how the blood that runs through our gums and teeth also travels around the rest of our body. We also discussed how inflammation from the mouth increases the chance of heart attacks and stroke. During this conversation, I explained my strategies to him, and he was sufficiently impressed to try them out for himself.

In his final year before retirement, Dr. Ron asked me to speak at his dental study club. He also told every patient in his practice about my method of oral care. He carefully explained the system to them. He soon noticed amazing results in the mouth health of his longtime patients. He reported shining teeth and greatly improved gum health.

Dr. Ron says that learning this kinder and more nurturing approach to mouth care was the most important thing he ever learned in dentistry, as its consequences far outweighed the benefits derived from implants, veneers, beautiful bridges, and other reconstructions he had done over his years as a clinician. This new approach allowed Dr. Ron to offer his patients a simple and effective method to reach a higher level of oral health. Dr. Ron urges other dentists to teach interested patients about these strategies and help them gain control over their dental problems. He says that, as a dentist, seeing such joy and empowerment will change your practice forever.

HEALTH SEEKERS

As we understand the link between mouth health and general health, the obvious problem is our inability to really know if our mouth is healthy. Visual observation or waiting for disease to develop can no longer be an acceptable method of mouth health evaluation. This also raises the importance of effective oral care and an evaluation of ineffective directions that many people have followed for years, often without any success. Perhaps the greatest confusion is in the minds of people who long ago understood the value of good bacteria—called probiotics—and their essential role in digestive health. I became a health seeker myself in the 1960s and learned the value of eating whole foods for health. I have avoided processed junk foods and toxic additives and have never consumed a can of soda in my life. I support the concern of health seekers about mercury in silver fillings, the toxicity from artificially fluoridating water, and the dangerous influences of some industries in their pursuit of profit.

The problem is that sometimes the truth is complicated, and we often don't know whom to trust. You may fear silver fillings and want to remove them, but be warned that white ones and sealants contain BPA, which may present its own dangers to your health. You may be against fluoridation of water as I am, but if your teeth need mineral support, as many do, the ideal helper is a tiny amount of sodium fluoride applied regularly to the outer enamel surface. Without this help, it is very possible that you will end your adult years simply suffering from different problems associated with root canals, crowns, and even losing teeth—damage that could have been prevented with a tiny drop of fluoride on the outside of your teeth.

If you are someone who needs to improve your mouth health, I hope you will consider a new approach that is kinder and more respectful of your mouth. The recommendations I share may seem simple and even mundane to someone who has endured years of pain and suffering. On the other hand, why not try a few weeks on my system and see what happens at your next dental appointment? My suggestions may be simple, but if you are looking for a different outcome, I encourage you to give them a try.

CHAPTER 3

Improving Your Mouth Health

*We stand at the proverbial crossroads. We have medicines
and practices that have served us well but have had
unintended consequences. . . . The practices that endanger
our children are at the core of modern health care.*

—Martin J. Blaser, MD, *Missing Microbes*

Many people have never contemplated their teeth, and only a few know
they are alive. Inside a tooth's thin outer shell are layers of living tissue
that contains cells, lymphatic liquids, and a network of blood vessels that
link directly to the blood flowing around our body. The outside of teeth
may feel hard to your tongue, but teeth are not a row of indestructible
pebbles. In fact, the best description may be that they are like a coral reef,
covered in delicate crystals that are nurtured or damaged by the saliva
and liquids that flow around them, in the way that ocean waters flow
around and influence the health of a coral reef.

Mouth bacteria are a big part of the mouth's ecosystem, and the
good ones help keep the mouth healthy. Similarly, saliva delivers minerals to teeth, but not if saliva is acidic, too viscous, too diluted, or sparse.
Like the ocean swirling over a coral reef, everything we eat, drink, or
put in our mouth becomes mixed with saliva and circulates to help or
harm teeth and influence the mouth's ecosystem. Drinks are particularly
influential. Even water dilutes saliva and makes it thinner and less able to
support tooth health, which is why we must consider the effect of meals
and snacks but more importantly the *frequency* of eating and drinking.
Everything that enters our mouth can affect saliva's pH levels and potentially improve or damage the mouth's ecosystem. Other influences we

need to consider are the drying and acidic conditions that are caused by mouth breathing and influences from the products we use to care for our teeth on a daily basis.

DETERMINING MOUTH HEALTH

In the United States, many people think they have good teeth. Their arbitrary assessment is often based on the fact that they have not had cavities in a while, or they simply think their teeth look good. Fillings, crowns, root canals, and implants are repairs for problems that are usually caused by dental disease. How do you know if your mouth remains infected or if it is getting healthier or less healthy? And how do you know if your tooth enamel is getting stronger or weaker? Any softening or sensitivity should be a red flag, because it shows minerals are leaving your teeth faster than they are being replaced. Excessive mineral loss is the cause of tooth sensitivity, which should be recognized as your teeth crying for help. Sadly, sensitivity pastes artificially block these important symptoms without addressing the underlying mineral imbalance, as they "fix" the symptom but ignore the underlying *reasons* for sensitivity.

Refusing to recognize gum disease is a problem for many patients. For years, gum disease has been tolerated or ignored in the United States, and detailed diagnosis of periodontal pockets has only recently become part of the routine at dental examinations. Gum pockets and periodontal disease are usually painless, and many dentists trained in the 1980s and 1990s were never taught how to identify this disease, despite the fact we have long known the damage that gum disease can cause and its potentially catastrophic impact on health. This situation is changing, and more physicians are now aware of the link between gum health and bodily health, although many do not understand how to advise patients who want to improve their home care. Be aware that, when dentists or physicians discover pathogens, they will usually want to prescribe antibiotics, strong antiseptics, or bleach combined with more frequent and deeper cleanings. My advice is to empower yourself and consider how you can first improve your mouth health with effective home care and potentially avoid antibiotics and aggressive strategies.

Many people assume they have a healthy mouth because they eat a good diet, exercise daily, and visit their dentist at regular intervals. When they experience cavities or gum disease, it can be shocking and make them feel angry, confused, or even depressed. If you consider the AAOSH Challenge results described in the preface, you will remember that even conscientious dentists had unhealthy periodontal pathogens in their mouths. This is why it is a good idea for anyone over the age of ten to have their saliva checked and, if they discover high levels of pathogens, begin using strategies to balance and control them to reach acceptable levels. Many of my clients have seen drastic improvements and a reduction in all their pathogens by simply following my recommendations for twelve weeks.

Good Mouth Bacteria

A healthy mouth is populated by a diverse variety of bacteria, and the broader this diversity, the healthier the mouth appears to be. In contrast, an unhealthy mouth will usually have a sparse and limited variety of bacteria, characterized by high levels of a few dominant pathogens. Current studies indicate that about ten billion bacteria live in the mouth, on teeth, on gums, and on the surface of the tongue. The Human Microbiome Project is focused on investigating these microbial communities and documenting how they influence health and the development of disease. This project reveals there are at least nine hundred strains of healthy mouth bacteria and that they have integrated systems to cooperate and communicate with each other, working in a harmonious way to protect our mouths from mechanical, chemical, and thermal damage.

In a healthy mouth with a wide variety of bacteria, there are usually about thirty to seventy families or *species* that are slightly more dominant than the others. Mouth bacteria float in saliva and move around until they find a habitat or location that will support their needs. This method of bacterial migration is called *colonization*. The dominant bacterial species in any mouth will therefore have a strong influence, and the most prevalent bacteria, be they good or bad, will usually determine the mouth's overall health. In the late 1970s, we learned that dominant mouth bacteria are most often the kind or strain that is the first to gain access and colonize occlusal grooves in molar teeth, areas that provide stable footholds for these bacteria, nestled in the anatomy of the tooth's flat biting surface.

In contrast to the nine hundred kinds of healthy mouth bacteria, there appear to be only about twenty bacteria that cause problems and can become destructive and harmful when they multiply. Some of these harmful bacteria are adapted to colonize teeth, but the majority, and some of the most destructive, breed in the depths of gum or periodontal pockets. The most infamous of mouth bacteria is a wild strain from a species called S.mutans. These bacteria have specific needs and flourish in acidic conditions, especially when they are undisturbed and are attached to a hard surface on which they can multiply. *S. mutans* are sticky by nature, and the firm, nonshedding platform of a tooth provides them with a perfect location to form thick layers, especially when they are able to feed frequently on sugar or carbohydrates in our diet.

Sometimes, the bacteria that live collectively in a defined space will be referred to as a *bacterial flora*. Our mouth flora can be imagined as resembling a flower-garden ecology. Weeds represent the harmful bacteria; flowers and grasses represent the beneficial ones. This analogy explains why aggressively clearing or stripping away weeds with harsh chemicals may remove weeds and clean up the garden, but it will also uproot good flowers and grass, which is why this not the best way to cultivate a healthy garden. Without nurturing healthy vegetation, a barren ecology will quickly become a home to more weeds, which may become even more invasive.

A healthy mouth needs a lush landscape with a wide variety of healthy bacteria that blend with each other and thrive with minimal care. This should be the goal for our mouth's ecosystem, especially since many bacteria offer us health benefits, especially the ones that grow in the grooves of molar teeth in healthy mouths. These healthy bacteria produce enzymes that are important because they initiate the digestive processing of gluten and carbohydrates in the foods we chew. Blocking molar grooves with plastic sealants, fillings, or artificial crowns removes this natural habitat and potentially decreases the population of these bacteria and the digestive help they provide. Helpful bacteria losing their habitat to sealants could be at least partially responsible for gluten or carbohydrate intolerance, weight gain, and digestive issues, and this concern must become a research priority before we seal all the molar grooves of children in America, which is the mission of the American Academy of Pediatric Dentistry.

BACTERIAL TRANSMISSION

Healthy saliva washes over your teeth and gums and carries many bacteria floating in it. These *planktonic microbes* are a mix of all kinds of bacteria, including kinds that are healthy and some that are potentially pathogenic. Saliva facilitates the bacterial transfer from one tooth to another in your mouth and also from person to person as you kiss your family members and share food. A baby's mouth is quickly colonized as soon as the first baby tooth erupts, and this occurs as bacteria travel and are shared from the mouths of people who interact closely or frequently with him or her.

Baby and adult molar teeth share a similar anatomy with crinkled biting surfaces. As soon as these teeth erupt, bacteria will colonize all the tooth surfaces and occupy every crevice, pit, and fissure to gain a foothold in an ideal location where they will become the dominant bacterial strain in a young child's mouth. Baby molars erupt before a baby is two years old, and adult molars erupt around age five. Droplets of saliva transfer as we talk and share food, cups, straws, silverware, or toothbrushes. Bacteria transfer from spouse to spouse; between siblings; among friends at school, babysitters, and caretakers; and even from the mouths of pets to their owners. Bacterial transfer may sound scary at first, but it is how a baby's mouth and body health is gradually strengthened. It is important to understand that having a wide diversity of healthy bacteria in your mouth will be healthful for you. In correct mouth conditions, these microbes will develop into a strong network and be able to protect your mouth from cavities and gum disease. This is why we should embrace bacterial transfer to a point and avoid the use of too many damaging antiseptics, antibiotics, and disinfectants whenever possible.

Infection on Toothbrushes

Unsanitary toothbrushes are a contributor to poor oral health, and I believe they may have played a much greater role in the explosion of tooth decay than has ever been considered. Today, we know toothbrushes pick up mouth bacteria during a single use. This may not be a problem if you have a healthy mouth, but it makes sense to be concerned if your family members have cavities or gum disease.

In New York, a state-mandated program in preschool and kindergarten classrooms insists children brush their teeth after lunch. The problem is that classroom brushes are often stored together in a large box or bag, potentially spreading infection from the children with cavities to those with healthy mouths. It seems equally wrong to suggest to communities or patients with poor oral health that a toothbrush per se will be helpful. There are superior ways to protect teeth from cavities, and toothbrushes have enormous potential to spread dental disease. Studies on toothbrush contamination are shocking, because they show the ease of contamination and how bacteria breed in toothbrush bristles. Brushes pick up the entire array of mouth bacteria, viruses, yeasts, and fungi, and some of these microorganisms remain viable on brush bristles for 2–7 days if the brush remains damp.

A few studies have examined the efficacy of products for decontaminating brushes. During a 2001 study, the researchers were amazed to find that 70 percent of the brushes in their study were heavily contaminated after one use. Placing a cap over the brush head appeared to encourage virulent opportunistic pathogens, like one called *Pseudomonas aeruginosa*, a species of bacteria that is adapted to low-oxygen environments. This is important information for anyone who travels or keeps their toothbrush in a gym bag, drawer, or confined space.

In 2007, researchers investigated the contamination levels for new brushes compared with older, worn brushes to see if older brushes would trap more bacteria. Three well-known brands of toothbrushes with soft nylon bristles were used: a brush with an oval head, a brush with flat bristles, and a brush with an average head design. The researchers used many brushes of each type. Half of the brushes were worn against metal brackets, whereas the rest of the brushes were unused. All brushes were immersed in a solution of *S. mutans* for five seconds. The brushes were then rinsed with water, and the first bacterial count was taken. The count was repeated twice, with the brushes being allowed to air-dry between the tests.

Immediately after immersion, all the brushes were heavily contaminated. After eight hours, there was contamination on all the brushes.

After twenty-four hours there were varying levels of contamination on all the brushes. The researchers were surprised that there were differences in contamination among the brands and that these differences exerted an influence on the bacteria collected in the bristles. Even more surprising, the new brushes appeared to harbor more bacteria than the worn ones at every time interval. This study indicates how easily brushes become contaminated and that rinsing with water does not adequately decontaminate an infected brush.

If you have cavities or gum disease, brushing may dislodge infected plaque, but your brush will be contaminated with harmful bacteria, and so it must be disinfected before you use it again. I suggest twenty-four hours of air-drying any toothbrush, but I also suggest you decontaminate the bristles of your brush after each use by swishing the head of your brush in an essential oil rinse like Listerine®. Then rinse it with water, and allow it to air-dry in a clean environment away from any toilet contamination.

Never keep brushes in a drawer, inside a travel case, or under a plastic cap. Do not rely solely on UV sanitizers either as they may not be as effective as portrayed by their marketing. Even antibacterial toothbrushes need to be cleaned with some frequency, especially if you have an unhealthy mouth. Finally, be wary of reusing a brush after you have packed it during travel. Consider purchasing inexpensive brushes for travel and use them as throwaways. A ten-dollar investment can buy you a handful of brushes and may save you thousands of dollars in periodontal treatments in the years ahead.

DANGERS TO MOUTH HEALTH

Our mouth and teeth are always under attack from our eating and drinking habits and from things that abrade, heat, chill, acidify, or dry them. This is why it's important to limit snacking, especially with acidic or sugary foods or drinks, and to protect our mouth from acidity as much as possible. There are a few foods that may nurture the protective coating in our mouth known as biofilm, and there are some foods that offer some dental benefits and protection. Xylitol is one of the most convenient of these foods, and it works in various ways. It is especially useful in our modern diet, because it can quickly help control mouth acidity. Alkalizing the mouth to a pH of around 7.4 will not only promote healthy mouth bacteria but will also prevent post-meal demineralization of teeth and any potential acidic damage to healthy biofilm.

If you have cavities or gum disease, you have harmful mouth bacteria that have infiltrated and likely become resident in the biofilm of your mouth. Unless you make changes, these bacteria can cause ongoing damage for decades of your life, possibly forever. Frequent dental cleanings, however deep, cannot clear away these bacteria completely from your mouth. Antibiotics or strong antiseptics may eradicate bacteria, but they are not selective and do not prevent harmful ones from returning, sometimes more aggressively than before. It's nice to think your hygienist is *cleaning* your teeth, but the terminology oversimplifies the situation.

Mouth bacteria float in saliva, and the diverse mix is made up of residents from the mouth and other areas, namely the sinuses, nose, and throat. A dental cleaning cannot change your saliva, nor does it promote healthy mouth bacteria. To change your mouth's ecosystem requires strategies that limit mouth acidity daily and improve the quality of saliva that washes over your teeth. Too frequent cleanings can in fact be a problem, especially for someone with a dry mouth who may have difficulty maintaining or developing healthy biofilm. Frequent cleanings can make teeth sensitive and possibly more prone to cavities if the protective biofilm is cleaned away. If you lack saliva, you will lack the salivary proteins that are the foundation of biofilm, so you will have difficulty building back the mouth's basic protection after it has been stripped from your teeth. Fewer cleanings and using techniques to nurture healthy bacteria will be beneficial for you and will help you to restore comfort to your mouth.

Any aggressive antiseptic, like chlorhexidine, or the use of an antibiotic can abruptly kill all mouth bacteria (good and bad) simultaneously. This may give you short-term clinical improvements, but these products can damage the beneficial bacteria in your mouth and create new problems, like candida overgrowth, gum recession, tooth abrasion, or sensitivity. The best way to develop sustainable oral health is to gradually improve your mouth health little by little. Along this progressive journey, you should ask your dentist about your mouth health and if you *need* dental cleanings. When cleanings are no longer required because they are no longer necessary, you will know that you have achieved healthy, stable, and sustainable conditions in your mouth—something I call *ultimate* oral health.

Gingivitis: Initial Gum Damage

When the gum around a tooth is tight and healthy, there is no risk of a pocket forming and no place for low-oxygen disease bacteria to multiply. This is why some kind of incident is necessary to cause the gum to be stretched and lose its grip on your tooth. Usually this occurs if the gum is irritated and becomes swollen. This can be the result of injury, but often it follows a small infection in an area. A wounded gum will, like any wounded body part, swell and bleed, especially if the area is rubbed or pricked. You may notice your gum bleeds easily but not remember the incident that caused the harm, possibly some lodged or abrasive food, a flossing cut, or toxins from infected biofilm (plaque) that irritated the area. Quickly resolving this infection will end the condition, which is called *gingivitis*. If your gums bleed when you brush or floss, it is likely you have gingivitis.

Often, gingivitis occurs when your body's immune system is weak or compromised, such as during pregnancy, a period of stress, hormone fluctuation, menopause, or if your mouth is dry from the side effects of taking certain medications or using an asthma inhaler or antihistamine drug. When you notice bleeding, it is important to take action immediately to resolve this, since leaving gingivitis unchecked can allow the gum band to loosen and the door to open for the next stage of gum disease.

While we will discuss the specific strategies of my Complete Mouth Care System in chapter 9, here are some things you can do to support healthy gum tissue: Use xylitol gum or mints after every meal, snack, and drink to alkalize your mouth and support the development of healthy biofilm. You should also use a clean toothbrush and massage this area, especially around the site of bleeding. The idea is to stimulate circulation of blood and lymphatics in this area and recruit healing help from the nutrients that the blood flow will bring to the tissues. You should also try to ensure that you support your body's immune system by eating healthy foods, especially fruits and vegetables with vitamin C, and other foods that provide a good mix of nutrients to benefit wound healing. These simple strategies can resolve gingivitis easily and stop more serious gum disease from developing. If gingivitis is untreated for more than a few days, deeper damage can occur, and a gum pocket may form that is much more permanent and difficult to resolve.

Gingivitis affects at least one in seven adults, even in the mouths of people who routinely visit their dentist. Few people realize how easy it is to treat this condition with good brushing, attention to nutrition, and the use of my Complete Mouth Care System to support healing. If your gums bleed as you brush them, this is a signal to brush the area more thoroughly, not less, since the improved circulation you will create by brushing will help the swelling go away before any permanent damage happens to your gums.

If cold water makes your mouth sensitive when you brush, use warm water on your toothbrush. If brushing is painful, try to clean the area initially with gauze or a cloth, wiping and massaging around the teeth. Once the area is clean, it will begin to heal quickly. Most people avoid brushing when they see bleeding, but this is exactly the wrong thing to do as it allows more bacteria to accumulate in the area and gingivitis to progress into a disease that can cause tooth loss. If you have previously noticed bleeding gums but they stopped bleeding, this may not be a good sign. This could signal that gingivitis progressed and became the next stage, which is a painless, nonbleeding, more serious gum problem called periodontal disease.

Periodontal Disease

There are only a few kinds of mouth bacteria able to thrive in the narrow space between a tooth and its surrounding and supporting bone—a place called a gum pocket. These bacteria are collectively known as *periodontal pathogens*. These pathogens are aggressive and flourish anywhere they find seclusion and a low-oxygen environment. They cause harm to the gum fibers that connect the root of the tooth to the bone, and some of these pathogens can open up wounds on the inside of the gum pocket, which can potentially allow them to gain access into the blood and travel to distant areas in the body.

Periodontal pathogens have individual names, specific characteristics, and each kind appears to target one or more specific areas of our body. Most of them cause a low-grade chronic inflammation in the gum tissue where they multiply. This small nucleus of trouble below the gums can work like a burning ember, and as the inflammation or infection is distributed by blood, it can ignite far more serious inflammation elsewhere in the body. Periodontal pathogens adapt to low-oxygen environments, and eleven species have been identified and found in pockets around teeth. Some periodontal pathogens cause a low-grade infection in the gums, others cause erosions inside the pocket, and some produce toxins or poisons. All periodontal pathogens initiate a reaction from the body's immune system, and the body responds by sending fighting cells to the area in an effort to control them.

In most cases, the body's immune system is unable to overcome these periodontal attackers, and a chronic battle ensues. Unresolved, chronic gum disease can continue with progressive, ongoing destruction and attachment loss, until the jawbone dissolves in the area around the tooth, which allows the tooth to loosen and possibly fall out. These problems are hidden under the gums, but they are serious, even though they rarely cause any swelling or pain. Certainly the most dangerous consequences occur when invasive periodontal pathogens get into the blood or when they create sufficient inflammation to ripple from the mouth to other places in the body, which can put you at risk for a stroke or heart attack.

Periodontal disease has never hit the news headlines or been publicized, because it is an invisible disease that doesn't cause toothache, bleeding, swelling, or the pain of other dental infections. Shocking statistics indicate that half of the young adults in America today are heavily infected with periodontal pathogens before the age of thirty. It seems unfortunate that carriers of gum infection often do not know the dangers of harboring high levels of these pathogens or how they are transferred from person to person by kissing and close contact.

Periodontal disease used to be called periodontitis, and it was thought to be a gum problem caused by food particles that were allowed to accumulate around and between teeth when patients were "bad" about brushing or flossing. The theory was that this debris caused damage, which led to pocketing, and when the pocket became too deep to be cleaned by a toothbrush, cleaning became impossible, so the situation escalated to eventual tooth loss. This was why a "critical pocket depth" was determined to be the length of a toothbrush bristle: 4 millimeters. Once a pocket was greater than 4 millimeters, dentists believed you would not be able to clean your gums adequately, and the prescribed treatment was then to cut the gums and reduce the pocket depth to less than 4 millimeters, so the toothbrush bristles could once again reach the bottom of the pocket.

Cutting the gums was a painful process that removed several millimeters of gum tissue, and as it reduced the pocket depth, it exposed several millimeters of the tooth's root, which made teeth sensitive and look exceptionally ugly. Dentists did not know the bacterial nature of periodontal disease at the time and could not understand why this disfiguring process, called *gingivectomy*, never stopped the problems. No one knew about the transmissible nature of periodontal disease and that reinfection from the mouth of a spouse or friend was possible. People often used old infected toothbrushes after this surgery, sometimes keeping them for months and even years, never considering it a risk. Patients were usually blamed for inadequate mouth care, because nothing seemed to stop the disease, and these unfortunate people often ended up with dentures as their teeth fell out.

In 1978, Paul Keyes, a researcher working at the organization now called the National Institute of Dental and Craniofacial Research, caused a dental uproar when he suggested bacteria were to blame for periodontal problems in gum pockets. He suggested the revolutionary idea to stop cutting gums; instead, he applied a mixture of baking soda and hydrogen peroxide plus systemic antibiotics, creating a nonsurgical treatment for gum pocketing. Dr. Keyes was a trailblazer, but today we know more, and even this therapy was less than ideal, leaving patients with gum recession and sensitivity. Some dentists have built on Dr. Keyes's original concept but with strong mouth disinfectants, antibiotics, aggressive antiseptics, or surgical-type cleanings aimed at removing biofilm and killing bacteria along the side surfaces of teeth (this process is called *root planing*). Dentists usually find it difficult or impossible to believe a pocket can heal naturally without this treatment or imagine that hard debris under the gums can dissolve in the correct mouth conditions and go away without root planing or antibiotics.

Root Sensitivity after Gum Disease

We have discussed how gums hug the tooth tightly at the place where the root meets the part covered by enamel in a healthy mouth. This area is called the *cement-enamel junction*. Healthy gum tissue is like a tight elastic collar, and it grips the neck of the tooth at this location to keep bacteria, liquids, and food particles from going below the gum surface. This mechanism protects the tooth's root from any damage by acidic or abrasive foods that could harm its delicate surface.

A tooth's root is covered with a soft, porous material called *cement*, which offers a perfect surface texture for the attachment of microscopic hairs that span between the tooth and bone. But this surface is not a shield and is easily damaged if it is exposed to the mouth, which is something that may happen as your gum recedes down to the root of your teeth or if a pocket opens up and allows liquids in this area. When gum tissues are damaged or if the gum loosens, root cement can come in contact with foods and liquids in the mouth. With no protection from acidic assaults and temperature changes, these sensations can travel through the tooth surface in the root area and are often perceived as sharp or even excruciating dental pain.

Root sensitivity is most often a symptom of gum problems, but it is usually felt as radiating pain in teeth, especially as you breathe or drink something hot or cold. Tooth roots are not good candidates for fillings, and sensitivity toothpaste will only cause additional discomfort, including a furry feeling on your teeth or the sensation of a dry mouth. My suggestion is to avoid peroxide, whitening products, oil pulling, or baking soda, which may lead to recession. Sensitivity will disappear naturally as your gum and tooth health improves.

Dentin Problems

The center of a tooth is alive, and it is called the *pulp*. Pressure-sensitive cells called *odontoblasts* are located in the pulp, and they have extension arms that radiate from the pulp and traverse across the main part of the tooth that is called the *dentin*. The arms of odontoblast cells run inside a small hollow tube, known as a *dentin tubule*. The cell's arm floats in this tubule bathed in lymphatic fluid that is in osmotic balance with the chemistry of your body and blood. This fluid provides a transport system for minerals from the body to supply internal areas of the tooth, keeping them hydrated, pliable, and healthy. Any sensation that upsets an odontoblast will be communicated to the nerve cells in the tooth pulp. Nerve cells transmit the problem sensations to your brain, where they are interpreted as pain. You feel such sensations when an odontoblast senses that bacteria are attacking a tooth or sometimes during dental treatment. To clean and shape a tooth for a filling, a dentist will drill out damaged areas, and if the drill cuts dentin, part of an odontoblast's arm can be severed. This creates alterations in fluid pressure in the tubule and sends an urgent signal to your brain, where this is perceived as intense pain.

Odontoblasts secrete a material that solidifies to become new dentin, and this is a process that can repair the walls of their tubule, even decades after a tooth has erupted. This mechanism continues slowly over time, and the internal walls of dentin tubules thicken gradually as you age. In a crisis, the odontoblasts use this attribute to barricade and close off one or more tubules to stop bacteria from reaching the live center of the tooth. This defense mechanism can be extremely effective if decay progresses slowly, but it is unable to compete with a bacterial attack that occurs rapidly. Odontoblasts are unique, and they appear to have a vital role in tooth health. Sadly it is your friendly odontoblasts that are most damaged by peroxide and when you treat teeth carelessly with bleaching or whitening products or chemicals.

How do you know when tooth pain is telling you something serious or if it is sensitivity that can be reversed naturally? The rule of thumb is that a painful sensation that lasts fewer than two minutes usually indicates the problem is reversible. You should consider this pain as a warning, but the situation may not be a disaster. Usually, the longer the pain continues, the more serious it is. When tooth pain is felt as you press on a tooth, this is usually a call for more urgent dental help, as this kind of pressure is normally caused by fluids accumulating from a bacterial infection inside the tooth or an abscess in or around the tooth's root.

Over half of the US population is now suffering from tooth sensitivity, which should be a warning that we are being careless in the way we care for teeth. In most cases, this pain is probably reversible with kinder and more preventive home care. Of course, pain from an abscess or dead tooth is serious, and if you are in pain and unsure of the cause, make an appointment with your dentist. If you want to try to determine a little more about sensitivity, consider what may be causing the problem. Here are some questions to ask yourself:

When you feel pain from hot or cold—

- Is the pain immediate, as if directly on the outside of the tooth?
- Is the pain delayed, or does it persist for more than two minutes, with it feeling like a throbbing inside the tooth?

When you eat or drink—

- Does the pain appear to come directly after food or drink?
- Does the pain start as you begin chewing or when pressing down on the tooth?

When you look at your teeth—

- Do you have thin enamel or a groove at the sides of the gum, all along your back teeth?
- Do you have a piece of tooth missing, a large old filling, or a cavity (hole) in the area?

If you answer yes to the first questions in each grouping but not the second, the problem is generally reversible. Everyone with sensitivity should take preventive action, but if you gave affirmative answers to the second questions, your problems are more likely to be caused by infection—either in your gums or in a tooth—so you should seek treatment sooner rather than later. If a tooth dies, bacteria will invade the pulp, causing a buildup of fluid that creates pressure inside the tooth. Unless dental care relieves this pressure, it will eventually push into the bone, forming an abscess, which can be painful and dangerous.

Many people have embraced white fillings as an alternative to silver ones, but patients often experience sensitivity and pain from a white filling and wonder why this happens. Silver filling material is a paste-like metal that solidifies after it is packed into a tooth to become a block known as an *amalgam filling*. The shape of this filling block is critical and complex, and dentists need to follow defined engineering rules if the filling is to stay in place. White filling materials are easier to use, because they can be glued to teeth, and less engineering design is required. This seemed great at first, but dentists discovered these white filling materials often set hard before they were correctly positioned.

New materials have been developed that remain fluid until they are cured with a light beam. It was a perfect solution until dentists discovered that this light caused the filling material to pull away from the tooth surface and move toward the light. This problem produces tension on the adhesive glue at the base of the filling and causes it to stretch like chewing gum, pulling away from the tooth's dentin surface and then bouncing back each time the filling is pressed by eating or clenching. Constant stretching and pulling changes the fluid pressure in the dentin tubules and can upset the odontoblast cells, which notify you with a signal that is felt as pain.

Fortunately, the Academy of Biomimetic Dentistry (ABD) has worked tirelessly to perfect placement techniques for white fillings and has taught ABD members how to properly adhere fillings, and they also teach a method where the filling is cured outside the mouth with a technique called *CEREC*. This group of dentists has also developed excellent methods to harden white fillings incrementally, sometimes interspersing and weaving fine mesh fibers between the layers to prevent any movement or shrinkage.

HEALTHY BIOFILM: A DEFENSIVE SHIELD

We've discussed how the mouth is home for hundreds of different kinds of bacteria, yeasts, fungi, and viruses—an invisible garden of life. The irony is that the healthiest mouths have the widest diversity of bacteria, and unhealthy mouths are dominated by a few aggressive and destructive kinds. In a healthy mouth, beneficial bacteria are woven into an invisible unit by thread-like strands of protein that form a transparent microfabric known as *biofilm*. The characteristics of a healthy biofilm are poorly understood, but it is more complex than the sum of the qualities exhibited by each individual bacterium that comprises the biofilm. For example, temperatures and chemicals that would harm individual bacterium subjected to a particular challenge suffer no harm or damage when they are meshed together as part of this biofilm. Two teeth in your mouth can host completely different bacterial species, but their communication systems, called *quorum sensing*, allow them to work in harmony and function as a coordinated unit to protect your gums and teeth in a powerful way.

A healthy tooth requires healthy biofilm to cover its surface if it is to attract minerals from saliva to enter into the tooth's surface. Healthy biofilm also acts as a shield, offering protection from thermal damage, from hot or cold food and drinks, from infection by invader bacteria, and from chemical or mechanical damage that could wear away the tooth's surface. Teeth devoid of biofilm will usually be easily weakened, more sensitive to hot and cold, more likely to decay, and more at risk for erosion and abrasive damage.

The first bacteria to land on a clean tooth will immediately begin to attract other bacteria and develop into tiny communities called *colonies*. The speed and type of colony that develops appears to be influenced and depend on the surrounding environmental conditions and by the type of bacteria that are first to initiate the colony. This happens because certain bacteria attract other specific kinds that may not be from the same family but appear to flourish in similar areas. This means we see certain kinds of bacterial groups in specific mouth neighborhoods, and these bacteria—good or bad—grow in numbers and become dominant. Acidic conditions, especially in mouths where sugar and carbohydrates are consumed, will promote aggressive cavity- and plaque-forming microbial communities, whereas alkaline conditions in mouths where carbohydrates and sugar consumption are controlled will promote a protective collection. Each colony is unique, yet through cellular communication they are never isolated, and they touch and interact with adjacent communities in every dimension. This is why bacteria in your mouth are biologically connected to biofilms that extend into other areas of your body.

The bacterial communities in your nose, for example, communicate with adjacent bacteria in the throat and sinuses. This is why children with plaque and cavities may also have frequent middle ear infections, postnasal drip, sinus problems, and even lung infections. As mouth health improves, the health of these adjacent areas may improve as well. This also means it's important to consider nasal and sinus health if you are trying to improve your teeth.

Healthy biofilm protects your mouth from all kinds of damage, but biofilm can become infected if changes tip its bacterial balance and the environmental conditions offer more support to harmful microbes. Things that can tip the health of biofilm are acidity, high-carbohydrate or sugary diets, any mouth-drying conditions (including medications), challenges to the immune system, prolonged illness, chronic depression, chemotherapy, or poor digestive health. The most common bacteria to infect oral biofilm are *S. mutans*, which can change healthy biofilm into a sticky mass in less than three weeks of unhealthy conditions, especially when accompanied by improper mouth care. These invisible microbes inflate the biofilm and can expand it until it becomes a foamy mass that is visible in the mouth as a material commonly referred to as *plaque*.

S. mutans bacteria attach to a tooth's surface by strands of a stringy, adhesive material they produce when they feed on carbohydrates and sugars from the foods we consume. These adhesive strands help *S. mutans* bind closely to the tooth's surface and to each other, forming blankets of tube-shaped bacteria that layer one sheet on top of the next. In this way, the sticky mass covers the tooth surface and it grows upward and outward. As the bacteria multiply, they form acids, which collectively acidifies the entire mesh of biofilm in which they are lodged.

Sugar and carbohydrates energize the bacteria of infected biofilm and make it grow rapidly and produce more acids. To the eye, this thick mass is often seen as a cream-colored material close to the gumline or in other sheltered areas between your teeth. The acids in this infected biofilm damage the tooth surfaces in any areas where it is attached, and the greatest damage occurs on surfaces exposed to acids for the longest time. When plaque remains undisturbed for several days, these acids will remove minerals from the underlying tooth and leach into saliva to weaken teeth everywhere in your mouth. Generalized mouth acidity is particularly dangerous, since it encourages the growth of a particularly aggressive type of bacteria that secretes poisons called *toxins*. These toxins irritate the gums and cause gingivitis and bleeding around the margins of your teeth.

When plaque is visible on your teeth, it is already seething with harmful bacteria. The more infected it becomes, the more puffed up it will be. Eventually, this infected biofilm can become thick enough to be scraped from teeth as a white, foamy slime. An infected biofilm that grows more slowly can be equally problematic, since it can calcify and thicken as it absorbs calcium and phosphates, and this will create a hard, crusty product known as *calculus* or tartar.

One kind of bacteria, *Corynebacterium matruchotii*, occurs in certain individuals' mouths and can increase the speed of calculus formation. These bacteria form a backbone or post-like structure, which becomes a support for bacterial film to grow more rapidly than in most other people's mouths. People who have a rapid buildup of calculus should avoid acidity as much as possible by eating and drinking at mealtimes and ending meals with xylitol or something that can alkalize the mouth. Before a dental cleaning, try to balance your mouth ecology with xylitol, improved nutrition, and careful eating patterns. Many people struggle with their digestive health, and this has an influence on mouth health. My suggestion is to supplement with a digestive probiotic for a few weeks before and after your dental cleaning. You need to support these probiotics by eating a wide variety of vegetables as part of every meal. A healthy digestion will improve saliva quality and this, in turn, will encourage the development of healthy bacteria and their supporting biofilm in the mouth. Eventually good bacteria will crowd out plaque-building ones, but this transition is progressive and may take months or sometimes longer. The key is to realize that we must begin with *digestive health* as it is the only way to improve saliva quality and unlock a lifetime of *sustainable* oral health.

Healthy biofilm appears to contribute many general health benefits as it protects the integrity of your cheeks, gums, teeth, tongue, and overall mouth health. Removing healthy biofilm removes this special protection and can leave your mouth and teeth vulnerable to damage. Without healthy biofilm, the mouth and tongue may be more prone to ulcers, sloughing, and soreness, and teeth are more easily damaged, thinned, and eroded, leaving them sensitive to temperature changes.

Each of us has a unique biofilm fingerprint that has developed over our lifetimes, incorporating all kinds of bacteria into the mesh that forms from our unique salivary proteins. The composition of biofilm is usually well developed by age five and may remain mostly unchanged over the course of our lives. The only caveat is if biofilm is removed or is frequently influenced by mouth acidity or dryness, by taking antibiotics or by the use of products that damage its biology or chemistry. For example, you may be surprised to learn that biofilm can be seriously harmed by "plaque control" or "whitening" pastes that contain damaging abrasive or caustic ingredients like peroxide, which can destroy the protein matrix of healthy biofilm. Unexpected damage can happen suddenly or slowly, and even an apparently static biofilm that has offered your mouth ideal protection for many years can be rapidly changed by modifications in the products you use, your health, or your lifestyle—things like eating more often, different food quality or acidity, or the introduction of snacking or sipping between meals.

Once a healthy biofilm has developed, it should be respected and protected, as we need its protection for our mouth and teeth. Removal of healthy biofilm will leave teeth unprotected, and this may make your mouth feel uncomfortable, sensitive, or dry, and it can cause a bad taste or make your mouth feel slimy. During a professional dental cleaning, healthy biofilm is removed by the traditional process of cleaning teeth with pumice or abrasives. This is why you may want to ask in advance if you *need* a cleaning and opt not to have one if the answer to your question is "no." A doctor's prescription for antibiotics, perhaps for some unrelated infection in a distant part of your body, can also damage healthy biofilm in your mouth. In addition to reducing the number of cleanings and avoiding antibiotics whenever possible, I also suggest you avoid baking soda and peroxide, because these popular products can be problematic, especially if you have a dry mouth, a delicate digestive system, or protein-deficient saliva.

Developing Healthy Biofilm

My desire is that everyone should be able to enjoy natural and pristine teeth and gums, untouched by dentistry—for a lifetime. This is often seen as a laughable goal by dentists who usually see teeth deteriorate with age and may have never witnessed cavities and gum disease reversing. The process of breakdown and rebuilding our body's skeleton is understood as a natural process that helps to keep our bones dense and healthy. There is a similar ebb and flow of minerals in and out of the outer layer of tooth enamel to maintain the health of teeth and basically keep them young and strong. Mouth health improves rapidly when two simple things are in balance: (1) when enamel breakdown is controlled by limiting mineral loss from acidic damage or mouth dryness and (2) when mineral deficits are replaced quickly and completely after any damage. When the amount of damage and repair are equal or if there are greater amounts of minerals deposited in teeth each day, a cavity cannot form, since as many minerals are entering the enamel as are leaving it. When extra minerals are provided to teeth regularly each day, any enamel weaknesses will slowly become more fully mineralized, cracks will heal, and the tooth should lighten in color naturally. During this process, any cavity will begin to repair and may even disappear completely.

This is why it is important to control prolonged periods of mouth acidity, and this may involve reducing habits like snacking, frequent sipping of drinks (even water), and allowing chronic stress to dominate your life. It is equally important to nurture the healthiest possible biofilm, ideally by keeping your mouth bathed in healthy saliva as much as possible. The health and pH of saliva is affected by diet, stress, changes in hormones and circulation, smoking, and the quality of nutrients absorbed from your food, which depends on the health of your digestive system. A mouth that is bathed in mineral- and protein-rich saliva will have the attributes and proteins necessary to form the foundation of a strong biofilm, which will provide an essential base for the absorption of minerals into teeth. These minerals that are absorbed into the outside of teeth are able to diffuse through the teeth and be used for natural repair and prevention of weak enamel and cavities. Minerals from saliva are attracted to a tooth by an ionic charge on the outside of it, and this charge, which is almost like a magnetic force, pulls the minerals toward and then into the tooth's surface. The caveat is that this only happens in the presence of healthy biofilm and when the mouth is at a neutral or slightly alkaline pH.

After a tooth has been cleaned, healthy saliva will immediately coat its surface with proteins and form a hydration layer that protects the outer enamel crystals. This protein layer has a great influence on the amount and type of minerals and bacteria that are attracted to the tooth's surface. Certain kinds of bacteria will be promoted, others will be rejected, and additional types of bacteria will be preferentially encouraged to join the developing community while others will be repelled from this developing community woven between the protein mesh.

In 2014, Dr. Erica Shapiro Frenkel of Harvard University and Dr. Katharina Ribbeck published a study in *Applied and Environmental Microbiology*, suggesting that bolstering the mouth's salivary defenses may be a better way to fight cavities than relying on sealants and fluoride treatments. These researchers noticed that when the saliva proteins called *mucins* covered teeth, they had powerful abilities to manipulate microbial behavior and prevent cavity-forming bacteria from attaching to the teeth and causing cavities. In healthy biofilm, bacteria woven into the mesh contribute and communicate within their network, with positive and negative interactions between members of the community. Healthy saliva and biofilm promote the mineralization of teeth. Your gums will become healthy when your mouth no longer supports the bacteria that grow into thick plaque and produce toxins that cause gingivitis.

Many dentists despair and are frustrated, because they believe patients do not brush or floss adequately, and this is often a charge leveled at patients who are unable to develop healthy biofilm with their current oral care methods. Sometimes their dentist may suggest stronger toothpastes, more frequent cleanings, or even antibiotics, but these products and methods are aimed at killing mouth bacteria, a problem that could easily send someone's mouth into an ever-deteriorating cycle.

My approach may be the answer for you, if you have been unsuccessful with your oral health and if you want to enjoy the oral health you deserve. My strategies work to nurture and develop healthy saliva and biofilm by focusing on the development of the following:

- Healthy mouth bacteria and saliva and the development of healthy oral biofilm
- Supportive home care and habits to fully mineralize your teeth
- Improved digestive health to maximize absorption of nutrients from foods for the support of your immune system (i.e., your defense from disease)

- The consumption of a diverse whole-food diet (about 80 percent plant-based) to support digestive bacteria and provide the nutrients necessary for dental and salivary health

In addition, your choice of oral care products is vitally important. Many products can be problematic, and even some apparently healthy choices can have a negative impact. There are many features to consider, and if you have been loyal to a homemade toothpaste recipe, but your teeth and gums are not comfortable and healthy, you may want to reconsider what you are using, since many oils, clays, salts, and glycerin can interfere with tooth mineralization. Other ingredients, like baking soda and peroxide, can dissolve salivary proteins and leave teeth devoid of their essential biofilm layer, making them sensitive and rough to the tongue. This will explain why some apparently healthy products may stop disease, but they allow different problems to occur, such as gum recession, enamel erosion, sensitivity, weakened teeth, and fractures. A mouth that is not comfortable is not healthy. My greatest concern is that some of these products, especially the pastes and rinses that are specifically designed to strip biofilm, may allow viruses, chemicals, bacteria, or free radicals to damage skin cells in the mouth, working as precursors for oral cancer.

HEALING MOUTH TISSUES

If you have chronic health problems, you may show signs of inflammation, and your doctor may have discovered elevated levels of C-reactive proteins in your blood. Anyone who is trying to lower these levels should consider the impact of oral health on chronic systemic inflammation. Healing gum disease is similar to healing any wound, and this process is dependent on help from your body's immune system. This is why anyone with gum disease must pay attention to their digestive health, the powerhouse that supports their immune system.

My clients work to improve their digestive health in a variety of ways. We consider foods, eating patterns, the use of colon probiotics (sometimes with additional digestive enzymes), and usually some vitamin and mineral supplements, at least for a limited time. Often, our body requires extra nutritional support to improve its chances of healing chronic health problems. I rarely recommend oral probiotics, which are probiotics targeted for the mouth. A healthy biofilm makes the addition of new bacteria difficult or impossible in the mouth, so oral probiotics will be of little use. On the other hand, oral probiotics can be useful in specific and extreme situations; for example, when people struggle with the development of healthy biofilm because they have a very dry mouth, are recovering from cancer treatments, or are in situations where their immune system is compromised and their mouth needs help. Regular use, along with xylitol at the end of meals and before bed, can help these patients greatly. It is important to check the quality of oral probiotics very carefully. Many are lozenge-type but are sweetened with harmful artificial sweeteners, including sucralose, which will negatively affect your digestive pH and potentially disrupt your digestive bacteria. You really want to try and find oral probiotics sweetened with xylitol if possible, since xylitol provides nutrition for these healthy bacteria to support them. Please check my website for more information about probiotics and products that my clients have found useful. When a good combination of supportive efforts are used for twelve weeks, most people notice changes in their saliva health, oral biofilm, and the health of their teeth and gums.

NEW UNDERSTANDING ABOUT ORAL HEALTH

This shift in oral health thinking is about developing a new awareness and respect for the community of helpful bacteria that support our mouth's health. For many years, dentistry has tried to meticulously clean teeth, often with sharp instruments, powerful antiseptics, and even antibiotics, thinking that the eradication of plaque will somehow mechanically "clean" your mouth and keep it healthy.

Healthy biofilm can be our mouth's best friend, but it is easily weakened by periods of mouth dryness, a variety of medications, antimicrobials, strong fluoride treatments, and even antibiotics taken to heal other parts of the body. If you have a balanced and healthy mouth, a strong biofilm is providing your teeth with an effective shield against sensitivity, staining, and cavities. Biofilm is your mouth's natural defense from abrasion and erosion, two problems that can occur while brushing your teeth or grinding your teeth. Instead of buying a new brush or a bite guard, maybe first consider why you may have lost the protection of your natural healthy biofilm, and do what you can to restore it.

Many people have used my strategies and have completely resolved gum pockets without deep cleanings or any surgical therapy. I never prescribe chlorhexidine, peroxide, or strong antibacterials, as these can kill all the bacteria in your mouth. Chlorhexidine is particularly dangerous, because it can create a lethal allergic response.

Your dentist may want you to have a deep cleaning, laser treatments, bone grafts, irrigation, or use of special toothbrushes, strong antiseptic, or antibiotics rinses for your periodontal problems. I suggest that before you begin any of these potentially expensive treatments, you should consider an inexpensive at-home alternative for at least a few weeks. A few simple strategies could improve your mouth health and reverse some or all of your periodontal problems with minimal fuss and bother. You may be able to surprise your dentist, because the program I recommend will address the low-oxygen periodontal pathogens but will preserve the healthy bacteria that help establish mouth health and pocket healing.

Healing in the mouth occurs in exactly the same way as healing occurs elsewhere in the body. Healing is not possible until a wound is free of the infecting bacteria, and this explains why, in a diseased mouth, dental problems have caused so much frustration and confusion. Few dental strategies remove the offending infection without killing the bacteria that are necessary to establish mouth health. My epiphany occurred years ago, and for decades, I have focused on nurturing the mouth health of my patients before we pursued any proposed treatment plan. I often notice that damage can regress and may even disappear, almost miraculously, when you use this approach.

This is why I believe it is good, if possible, to implement my strategies and begin developing and maintaining healthy biofilm *before* you decide to have fillings, deep cleanings, or other treatments. Why not make improvements for a few months and use my Complete Mouth Care System, which we will explore in chapter 9, before you schedule your next dental cleaning? You may not be able to eliminate this first cleaning, but your improved state of mouth health will set you up for more success in the future and maybe help you to extend the intervals between cleanings, something that will only be possible if your mouth health improves.

CHAPTER 4

Nutrition for Oral Health

Eat food. Mostly plants. Not too much.
—**Michael Pollan**, *Food Rules: An Eater's Manual*

There is no doubt that supporting our body with quality nutrition and smart eating habits is a cornerstone of health. As a dentist, I am excited about the pentose non-sugar sweetener called xylitol, because it offers a powerful tool for improving tooth and mouth health, but it is also a great, but poorly understood, contributor to our digestive and general health. Xylitol stabilizes blood glucose levels, is helpful to diabetics, provides fiber and butyrate for digestive health, and can also positively influence nasal, sinus, pharyngeal, and potentially bone health. Most people are aware that many foods contain nutrients that offer us health benefits. Many of these foods are acidic, and I am often asked how to eat healthy foods like citrus fruits or drink liquids like cider vinegar, which are good for the body, but which are sufficiently acidic to cause erosion and damage to our teeth. In this chapter we will discuss how nutrition affects oral health and how to consume potentially tooth-damaging, yet healthy foods, without causing dental erosion or other damage.

As a teenager in England, I was very aware of nutrition, and I joined the whole-food movement of the 1960s, which taught the importance of diet for good health. I learned about the benefits of consuming certain foods, and I became convinced that a diet centered on natural foods, including whole grains, live-culture yogurt, nuts, fruits, and vegetables, could promote health. I read books about food science and followed health gurus who taught Eastern medicine and the benefits of adding herbs and spices to meals.

I have always valued a healthy diet, but I think it may be shortsighted to imagine there's a one-size-fits-all specific food selection for everyone. I believe some foods may suit certain people and that our needs may change as we age or adopt different lifestyles over the years. Portion control, variety, and moderation make sense, but so does the inclusion of fermented, seasonal, and local foods and the addition of herbs and spices. Updated science indicates that our digestive ecosystem is quickly changed, directed, and dependent on the kinds of food we consume, so that the more limited and unnatural our menu, the more limited and less healthy will be the diversity of bacteria in our digestive tract.

I believe that for health we must find a way to satisfy our body's needs for all the proteins, vitamins, minerals, flavonoids, and phytonutrients that are necessary to sustain and repair our body. The worst diets for health were probably in the 1980s when people wrongly believed that artificial sugars and processed low-fat foods were good choices. Obviously, it seems wise to control sugar and carbohydrate consumption, but it may be more important to focus on enjoying nutritious food combinations in a relaxed meal format than to fear every ingredient or try to pinpoint one food and blame it for our health problems. We are discovering that foods have many oral and general health benefits, and when they are consumed in certain combinations, their benefits may be enhanced, or one food may offer protection from an ingredient in the other that could otherwise be a problem or cause digestive upset. Remember, eating should be about foods, not ingredients!

I work hard with my clients to improve their mouth health; this usually means we also need to address their digestive health. I believe poor oral health can contribute to poor digestive health and vice versa. As I work with clients, we try to add a wide variety of plant-based foods to their menu choices and often notice substantial improvement in their mouth health as this occurs.

Many people today eliminate entire food groups from their diet, worried that dairy products, for example, are problems for their digestion. I would argue that for health we may benefit from all the food groups, and I believe dairy products should not be grouped as one entity, since 20 ounces of poor quality skim milk in a latte should not be compared with 4 ounces of whole milk from grass-fed, hormone- and antibiotic-free, pasture-raised cows. For these reasons, I usually reintroduce small amounts of high-grade butter (for example, melted with cooked vegetables), even for people who believe they need to eliminate dairy. Once we have introduced butter successfully, we then try 2- to 3-ounce portions of organic, unsweetened yogurt, mixed and sweetened with a teaspoon of maple syrup or xylitol or 1 ounce of fresh pineapple or papaya to aid digestion and counter acid reflux problems.

THE INTERPLAY BETWEEN DIET, DIGESTIVE HEALTH, AND NUTRITION

Dr. Weston Price was a dentist who lived in the early 1900s, and he is known for his observations on how nutrition appeared to affect dental and physical health. Dr. Price is still revered for his work documenting the diet and habits of various cultures and their effect on mouth development and oral health. He, along with many others, concluded that diets with substantial amounts of refined sugar and flour cause deficiencies that result in dental and medical health problems, which can be compounded generation after generation if nutritional deficits continue.

Foods not only affect our general health, they directly influence our mouth's ecosystem in a positive or negative way as they are chewed and eaten. The more sugary and refined our diet, the more we feed the harmful bacteria and yeasts that use these sugars and carbohydrates to grow and form sticky plaque on our teeth. In a similar way, our diet affects the variety of bacteria in our digestive tract, for better or worse. We now know that the more limited and unhealthy our diet, the more limited and unhealthy will be our variety of digestive bacteria. High-carbohydrate diets can promote harmful bacteria, but a limited or deficient diet can also cause problems. This is because, without digestive bacterial diversity, we may consume healthy foods but be unable to adequately absorb nutrients from them. The body depends on good nutrition to heal itself, and our immune system can be compromised by an inadequate selection of supportive foods or by poor absorption of nutrients from healthy foods that are consumed, but not adequately digested. This can occur when we have poor digestive health or when there is a speeding up of the passage of food during digestion, something that can occur in times of stress or hormonal imbalance.

Healthy digestive bacteria, adequate stress control, eating slowly, *and* a good diet are essential for the absorption of nutrients into our blood and bodily fluids. These absorbed nutrients travel around the body and become incorporated into saliva, affecting its quality and healing powers of our teeth and gums. This is why, for optimal mouth health, we should try to nurture a wide diversity of digestive bacteria and eat a varied diet that includes a healthy selection of plant-based foods.

DIGESTIVE HEALTH AND ORAL HEALING

Any acidic or sugar-containing foods or drinks—even healthy ones like fruit—can damage teeth. You don't have to remove these healthy foods from your diet, because there is a simple way to overcome the negative effects of localized acidity in your mouth and enjoy the positive general health benefits these foods offer. Up to a point, we should embrace the mineral loss that happens when we are eating and drinking. Healthy saliva will quickly provide minerals to replace any that were lost, and the newly deposited minerals will actually help to keep our teeth shiny and strong. This is why good eating and drinking habits allow periodic mineral loss but the lost minerals are immediately replaced from saliva. This is why we must complete every meal with a drink or food that alkalizes the mouth and then give time for our saliva to interact with our teeth. With this approach, we can stop worrying and consume potentially tooth-damaging foods without concern.

Xylitol is my ultimate choice immediately after acidic exposures, because it stimulates a flow of mineral-rich saliva into your mouth to encourage this mineral repair.

Acid-Alkaline Balance

We've talked about erosive tooth damage caused by mouth acidity and the benefits of mineral-rich alkaline saliva for mineralizing teeth to keep them strong. Some people consider that a similar acid-versus-alkaline balance for general health and suggest specific foods believed to alkalize the body for this purpose. It is confusing that many of the foods and drinks that are recommended for body alkalizing are extremely acidic, with a low pH and the potential to cause substantial damage and erosion to your teeth. Lemon juice and apple cider vinegar, for example, can cause dramatic problems for your teeth, yet they can be great for health and boosting your immune system. So, the dilemma is how to benefit from these things while avoiding any damage in your mouth.

The ideal solution is to consume foods and drinks as components of mealtimes and to not worry about their pH or acidity, providing the final food in your mouth is something that is alkaline, such as a piece of cheese, celery, or xylitol. Andrew Rugg-Gunn, professor at the Human Nutrition Research Centre at Newcastle University, United Kingdom, has authored many studies showing the effects of food on teeth over the past twenty years. This pattern of eating allows you freedom to eat any food safely, but you always end the meal with a tooth-protective food.

FOOD PAIRING

Most people are aware that many of the foods we consume contain an abundance of vitamins, minerals, and other important health nutrients. A new science of food pairing shows that when we eat foods in specific combinations, we can increase their nutritional value to a level that is higher than the sum of eating them individually, which allows us to reap additional health benefits. Most combinations taste really good and encourage meal-style eating. For example, studies at Purdue University showed that by adding eggs to salad, we can increase our absorption of nutrients from the egg *and* the salad greens, compared with eating these foods individually. The study showed that adding three eggs to a salad increased the absorption of carotenoids from the vegetables by three- to nine-fold, compared with an eggless salad.

Other food combinations work by offering a way for minerals to be more easily absorbed, or they may nurture specific kinds of digestive bacteria. For example, bananas are a good source of inulin fiber, and inulin supports a kind of digestive bacteria that is responsible for increasing calcium absorption from the gut. When bananas are eaten alongside whole milk, custard, or yogurt, this combination increases the body's uptake of calcium from the dairy. Spinach is another food that can be paired to increase its nutritional value. Spinach is nutritious, but it contains oxalate, which is an acid with sufficient strength to pull calcium out of teeth and cause tooth erosion. Oxalate also interferes with your body's ability to absorb calcium from the spinach, since oxalates bind calcium. Adding some vitamin C, like citrus juice, can help block oxalates from binding with calcium, and light steaming can also reduce the oxalates in spinach and limit this effect while preserving the water-soluble minerals that would be lost in boiling water. To increase the absorption of fat-soluble minerals from spinach or other green vegetables, consider adding a small serving of butter to these foods.

Incidentally, the oxalates in spinach do not interfere with calcium absorption from other foods that may be eaten with spinach, but it does take fifteen or more cups of spinach to match the amount of calcium in a cup of milk, which means that relying on spinach for daily calcium may not be a good idea.

Vitamin C also helps increase the absorption of iron from meat, so it is good to serve vegetables high in vitamin C, like chili or bell peppers, kale, broccoli, and cauliflower as accompaniments to meat dishes. Similarly, the vitamins in strawberries and blueberries are better absorbed if they are eaten in combination with dairy (think about strawberries and cream) or alongside foods that are rich in vitamin E (such as almond, peanut, or sunflower seed butter), since vitamins C and E appear to have synergistic absorption benefits. These examples are just a few of the amazing new discoveries about food pairing for health.

Protecting Enamel

I have already mentioned one or two reasons why it is ideal to end meals with xylitol, but it's useful to know that certain other foods can also offer tooth-protective benefits. Some of these protective foods can be eaten alongside damaging acidic drinks or sugary snacks to help protect your teeth. For example, nibbling cheese will alkalize your mouth and help mineralize teeth between sips of acidic wine. Whole milk, but not skim milk, can protect teeth and help to prevent acidic damage, which makes it a useful drink alongside sugary products, like an occasional cookie or piece of cake. Snacking on fresh or nutritious dried fruits or drinking fruit juice may be delicious, but this can cause horrific tooth damage, because the sugars in these foods and drinks allow the mouth to become and remain acidic for an hour after every sip, snack, or meal. After drinking acidic or sugary juices or snacks, consider having some xylitol in the form of a mint or piece of gum, some cheese or a drink of whole milk.

Tooth damage depends on the *length of time* that the mouth is acidic. This is why nibbling a small sugary or acidic snack over time will create more damage than consuming a larger quantity in one sitting, or ideally as a component part of a meal. This explains why sipping—especially acidic juices, coffee, tea, sports drinks, or smoothies—can be so harmful. Instead, try to consume these foods and drinks as part of a meal, and at the conclusion, end with xylitol, a tooth-protective food, alkaline water, or milk.

A dry mouth or acidic saliva can make it even more difficult to regain a safe, alkaline state in your mouth after eating, and often post-meal acidity will continue to demineralize teeth for hours. The best endings for meals are tooth-protective foods, which also make the best dentally safe snacks. These foods include salty nuts, cheese, yogurt, alkaline vegetables like celery, avocado, nut butters, and protein foods, like chicken or turkey and, of course, one of the most convenient, xylitol.

FOODS THAT FIGHT PLAQUE

Many foods have been shown to have so-called antiplaque abilities, but this attribute should always be considered in context. Many of these foods and juices are very acidic, which should make you wary of thinking they offer any practical dental benefits. Cider vinegar or cranberry juice, for example, can severely erode tooth enamel. Also, we now have improved knowledge about the importance of preserving healthy biofilm, something that was never considered in older studies, where biofilm removal was often the goal. I have seen incredible damage in the mouths of people who used inappropriate products as ingredients in their homemade toothpastes and rinses. One lady eroded all her teeth and lost all her fillings by following the bad advice to rinse with apple cider vinegar. Remember that sensible habits and a healthy mixed diet are the fundamental supports for whole-body and oral health, not one magic paste, food, or rinse.

Many oral care products contain ingredients that have been touted to reduce or remove plaque. Even natural care products have used this approach and include oils, baking soda, clays, food extracts, and herbs that are known to eliminate oral biofilm. Remember, we need a foundationally new approach for oral health, and it can be confusing, because most of the old studies suggest that biofilm removal is a benefit. I only recommend products that are able to support the development of healthy biofilm, and I suggest that unless you are convinced a product is tooth-protective you should use it with great caution.

Cranberries, Green Teas, and Cider Vinegar

Cranberries are a food that can damage teeth, and their juice has been studied and shown to reduce plaque. Cranberry juice is extremely acidic, and it is often mixed with other fruit juices as a cocktail. If you were to swish cranberry cocktail or even plain cranberry juice, it could easily ruin your teeth by eroding enamel and *causing* demineralization. It's possible you have heard similar studies about grape seed extract, green tea, cider vinegar, and other foods that can reduce dental plaque, but I suggest these are completely inappropriate products for oral care.

Apples

Apples are widely believed to be food for oral health, and they do contain an antioxidant called quercetin, which has antimicrobial and anti-inflammatory properties. Apples also contain *polyphenols*, which offer specific protection against gum damage by periodontal bacteria. Eating apples can benefit teeth, but always remember that *apple juice* is damaging. The difference is that juice loses its fiber component, and it is the fiber that protects teeth from the malic acid that apples contain. The difference is that juice loses its fiber component, and it is the fiber that protects teeth from the malic acid that apples contain. This is why I recommend eating apples whole or shredded. Shredding apples is a simple method to make them easy to digest, yet keep them safe for teeth. If you give apple juice to children, this can cause rapid decay, so it should always be consumed during mealtimes, and followed with something tooth-protective like xylitol.

Tea and Coffee

Most teas contain polyphenols or *catechins*, and green tea has up to six kinds of catechins that have been found to remove dental plaque. Teas can also be acidic, and this is why sipping tea can strip your teeth of its natural protection and allow your teeth to demineralize and stain. Tea may be less harmful to teeth than juice or sodas, provided it contains no sugar or lemon, but avoid sipping tea for too long, and always end your teatime with a tooth-protective food or xylitol.

Coffee is acidic, and it also contains a chemical called trigonelline, which gives it an aroma and taste as well as antibacterial properties. Coffee may cause mouth bacteria to be less adhesive, and sipping it slowly can be a problem for teeth. My suggestion would be to consume these foods and drinks you enjoy at mealtimes and finish the meal with an alkaline food or xylitol to protect your teeth and gums from damage.

CARIOSTATIC FOODS

When your mouth is healthy, it will feel fantastic. You will quickly find that any snack, drink, or meal can take away this super-clean sensation. My recommendation is not to run for a toothbrush after eating but to dilute and balance mouth acidity as soon as possible, using xylitol or another cariostatic product that can help neutralize acidity and stimulate a flow of saliva to remineralize your teeth. *Cariostatic* describes a food or ingredient that can actually help stop cavities from forming. Here is a short list of some foods and drinks that help alkalize the mouth and offer tooth-protective and mineralizing benefits.

Chocolate

People have been very confused by the diet fads of the 1980s and often appear to fear good and nutritionally beneficial foods yet embrace things like diet soda or low-fat processed foods, thinking low-fat and diet products are healthy. I have always believed in whole foods and eating in moderation, and now many delicious and nutritious foods, including chocolate, have been shown to have general health and mouth-protective qualities.

The 1954 Vipeholm study by Gustafsson et al. showed that people at high risk for tooth decay could eat dark chocolate and have fewer cavities than people eating comparable amounts of sugar. In 1986, Japanese researchers found that cocoa beans contain an ingredient called theobromine, shown to have cavity-preventing abilities; today, some toothpastes contain this chocolate extract. Of course, some chocolate is heavily sweetened with sugar and other ingredients, so we must apply this chocolate information sensibly into our lives.

Milk and Cheese

One of the most cariostatic foods is whole milk, and whole-milk cheese can be consumed at the end of a meal to protect teeth from cavities. In a 1994 study by Gedalia et al., seven- to nine-year-old children ate a small five-gram piece of Edam cheese after breakfast for two years. At the end of the study, the researchers found significantly fewer cavities in these children than in the control group that did not eat cheese.

We know that milk contains a sugar called *lactose*, but the only bacteria that can convert lactose to lactic acid are very aggressive kinds of plaque bacteria that have become anaerobic. These specific bacteria can ferment milk, but they are found only in thick, infected plaque that has been stagnant for days. When we drink fresh milk with a healthy mouth, there is no concern. Milk pH is around 7.0, and whole milk contains many helpful fats and nutrients that are protective of teeth. Tooth damage from consuming something acidic or sweet can be mitigated by the calcium and phosphates in milk to reduce enamel damage, as shown in studies by M. E. Thompson et al.

Do not confuse whole and skim milk. The sugar content in skim milk is actually damaging to teeth. If you find whole milk too thick, try diluting it with water rather than using skim milk. This way the fat content remains balanced, and the benefits of whole milk will be preserved. The cream on the top of non-homogenized milk is one product that may stimulate or speed up the formation of healthy biofilm. Consuming or rinsing with this cream may help you if you have a sensitive mouth that may have been stripped of its protective layer by overzealous cleaning; if you have a dry mouth; or after whitening treatments or following oral damage caused by chemotherapy. Here's an added tip: If your tooth is knocked out in an accident, and you are unable to take it to a dentist for implantation, carry it in a container of saliva, saline solution, cream, or milk to keep it viable for implantation. The quicker this is done, the better!

The following ideas are core to the nutrition and lifestyle strategy I have used to improve mouth health for over thirty years:

- End every meal, snack, or drink with a tooth-protective food, such as xylitol.
- Maintain digestive health, and keep sugar and carbohydrates to a minimum.
- Use xylitol mints or gum each day in conjunction with effective mouth care products to nurture a healthy mouth ecology.
- Don't sip or snack constantly, but drink at mealtimes, and give your teeth sufficient time between meals to interact with your saliva, every day.
- Eat plenty of vegetables and salads to nourish your body with adequate minerals, and consider adding garlic, mushrooms, and onions to boost your immune system.
- Consider the importance of eating a variety of food-sourced vitamins, especially vitamin C and vitamin D.
- Get plenty of sunshine, relaxation, and exercise to support your immune system.

NUTRITIONAL SUPPLEMENTS

Followers of Weston Price's ideology figured out some decades ago that sugar had a negative impact on digestive health. They also knew that sugar was only part of the equation and that our body needs vitamins and minerals for healing. Many of these people were concerned about our standard American diet and believed it had become severely deficient in calcium, magnesium, and other vital nutrients necessary to sustain health. There are many theories and different strategies about diet, but most experts will agree on the value of eating real, wholesome foods and the need to include a wide variety from the plant kingdom. Nutritional science is now confirming the wisdom and benefits of this type of diet for superior health.

High-quality, food-derived vitamin and mineral supplements can be a bonus if you are trying to improve your health or if you are experiencing times of stress, especially if you are vegan or nearly vegan or if you eat a limited selection of foods for some reason. I guess, if we lived in a perfect world, supplementation would not be necessary, because we would derive all our daily nutrients from foods. Unfortunately, this may not be possible or practical for some people, and supplements can sometimes fill these gaps. I believe nutritional supplements have been a boon to my clients while they work to change their oral health from a bad state, hoping to make big strides and see rapid improvements. As you begin your journey to improved oral health, I suggest you start by viewing your digestive tract as a vital part of this healing equation and see the process as a kind of top-to-toe internal gardening venture. The strategy for health improvement begins by seeding as wide a variety of healthy digestive bacteria in your gut as possible, and this can be achieved by alternating quality digestive probiotic supplements with a diet rich with plant-based and fermented foods, which will support them. As healthy bacteria flourish, these need to be continually nurtured by a fiber- and vegetable-rich diet. The addition of butter also provides benefits, since butyrate can improve colon health and increase the absorption of nutrients from foods. To heal dental or gum issues and develop ideal oral health, you will need to consider dietary improvements as an addition to your daily oral care and acid-control strategies. Good nutrition can improve the mineralizing capability of your saliva, but this can take time (from weeks to years) to fully manifest, depending on how dysfunctional and damaged your digestive and immune systems have been in the past. You may already have tried to improve your digestive or mouth health, but be encouraged, because working on these areas *simultaneously* will be far more rewarding and will usually give great results.

THE NEED FOR GOOD BACTERIA

Teeth are a living part of your body, and we should think of them less as a row of stones and more like a coral reef, if we want a better image of why they require nurturing and adequate contact with healthy saliva. Saliva is naturally equipped to supply teeth with the minerals, hydration, proteins, and bacteria they need for health. The bacteria in your mouth live not only on your teeth but also on the skin of your mouth, tongue, and in the oral liquids that make contact with the lining of your nose, ears, and throat. Once we understand that the inside of our body is clothed with an ever-changing but unified ecosystem, it is easier to understand why our digestive, respiratory, and oral health can be either supportive or problematic for other areas of the body.

Today, we know that many microbes, fungi, and virus strains are normal residents in our digestive tract, and many are important contributors to our health. In the dynamics of this ecology, good bacteria usually help control harmful bacterial overgrowth, and there are some microbes that specifically stimulate and strengthen our immune system, the mechanism that controls our body's ability to repair wounds, fight infection, and detoxify our body to keep us healthy and alive. Achieving a healthy balance of microbes in our digestive tract appears to be central to our well-being and ability to heal.

To change your digestive health, I suggest you consider introducing some food-based vitamin and mineral supplements for a few weeks to support your new developing digestive flora. The direction of change is improved by limiting carbohydrates and sugars at this time and adding as wide a variety of plant-based foods as possible to your diet. If you decide to take probiotic supplements, I suggest you initially target your colon, but remember that all probiotics do not have equal effectiveness, and if you do not see digestive improvement within a few weeks, try using a different brand. It is always good if probiotics are tailored to your gender or age, and it is often good to ask advice from a trusted natural health food counselor or someone who is familiar with the latest research on this topic.

Fermented Foods

The words *probiotic food* have become synonymous with yogurt because of intense marketing by some yogurt companies. Don't be misled or let this taint your appreciation of probiotic foods, because there are an incredible number of fermented foods that can supply us with probiotic digestive support. Once again, use small amounts daily, and try to enjoy a varied selection. Fermented foods can be a fabulous addition to your diet if you are looking for improved digestive health. I encourage you to take steps and expand your horizons with fermented foods as you incorporate small amounts of the ones you like into your menu regularly. Here is a list of frequently used fermented foods in the United States:

- Brine pickles (kosher dill)
- Kimchi
- Sauerkraut
- Miso, tempeh, and natto
- Yogurt, kefir, and ryazhenka
- Raw-milk cheese
- Salami and other fermented, dry charcuterie
- Kvass and kombucha

Oral Probiotics

I encourage everyone to realize the importance of healthy oral biofilm and good bacteria in their efforts to naturally heal cavities and gum disease, but I do not generally recommend oral probiotic supplements, because a healthy mouth biofilm will reject new bacteria as intruders. In addition, dental problems usually start with an imbalance in the health of your saliva, and this should be your first focus to resolve tooth or gum problems. Most often, a poor quality saliva is the outcome from many years eating a poor diet or suffering from inadequate digestive absorption. You will not benefit in the long term by simply adding more bacteria to a basically unhealthy mouth. Oral probiotics may offer a temporary benefit if you are unable to improve your mouth health through diet and nutrition, but I suggest the first step for everyone is to develop a healthy pattern of eating and ensure you end every meal, snack, and drink with tooth-protective xylitol or other safe food to limit mouth acidity. Next, you should consider the system of oral care I share in chapter 9, but never think a single paste or rinse is all you need for a healthy mouth. This is why diet and good nutrition, possibly with the addition of nutritional supplements and digestive probiotics, fit into a well-rounded oral health program. The very last resort would be to try an oral probiotic, only if all the other steps have failed.

You should be shocked to know that some oral probiotics that are currently distributed through dental offices are sweetened with artificial sweeteners like sucralose and should be avoided. As mentioned, I recommend oral probiotics only as a last resort for someone who is unable to maintain mouth care or target his or her underlying problems. Look for oral probiotics sweetened with xylitol—included because xylitol feeds healthy, probiotic mouth bacteria. Oral probiotics may offer some help in dire circumstances or if you have an unstable mouth ecosystem because all the grooves in your teeth have been obliterated by dental crowns, fillings, or sealants. The fissures in molar teeth are vital places for healthy mouth bacteria to reside and gain a foothold, and without these footholds, you may have a more changeable mouth ecology and may also experience difficulties digesting gluten and carbohydrates, since these bacteria in molar fissures are primarily responsible for this digestive function.

NEW UNDERSTANDING ABOUT FOODS FOR HEALTH

In the 1960s, most people thought the digestive tract was a tube where food was processed to provide calories as our energy source. Counting calories was fashionable, restricting fat was supposed to be healthy, and if you were sick, doctors prescribed pills to destroy the illness-causing germs. My parents substituted saccharine for sugar and margarine for butter. If they felt slightly sick, the doctor prescribed one of the great new antibiotics or some other pill that they believed was able to miraculously make the sickness "go away."

Today, we look at these ideas in a new light and know the value of a correct mixture of microbes and that our health and energy are dependent on the work of healthy gut bacteria as they aid digestion and facilitate our body's absorption of nutrients from foods. These healthy bacteria in our gut have also been shown to influence our brain, our nervous system, how we feel, and even our body's response to infection and healing. In other words, healthy bacteria affect almost every aspect of whole-body health. This dramatic shift in understanding about our digestion has influenced what a healthy diet should look like and has underscored the importance of fermented, whole, and natural foods; healthy fats; and fiber to support the bacteria involved in the maintenance of our brain, heart, and digestive health. A similar shift now needs to happen as we think of mouth health, so we can move away from the misinformation that most people have believed for the past sixty years and begin to enjoy better oral health.

The Connection between Oral Health and Digestive Health

The most effective way to improve your oral health is to feed, nurture, and support good mouth bacteria and develop healthy oral biofilm. We can achieve this if we can control mouth acidity and improve the quality of our saliva, which is influenced by the nutrients we absorb and the health of our immune system. Body liquids travel in our lymphatic and circulatory systems, and these carry nutrients and cells everywhere around our body (including the tissues that surround our teeth), filtering into the saliva that bathes them. This is why our immune system exerts a big influence and why I advocate some surprising foods for mouth health, including garlic, mushrooms, carrots, onions, pomegranates, dates, and figs. These are wonderful foods to nourish, detoxify, and boost your immune system, which in turn will support the health of your gums and teeth.

Ask anyone in the naturopathic world, and they usually have great respect for healthy digestion, but they often overlook the importance of mouth health. As bacteria have been investigated and cataloged, biofilms have become a new interest, and new facts about them are coming to light and being documented by the Human Microbiome Project. This project has looked at bacteria on skin, in the digestive tract, and in the mouth. Each location appears to have its own kind of ecosystem, supporting special types of bacteria, and researchers have found similarities in biofilms, especially where they interconnect. For example, bacteria in the nose, sinus, ears, and throat are specific to each location, but they are influenced by the composition of bacteria in adjacent ecosystems. This illustrates why it's impossible to have good oral health if anatomically adjacent areas are unhealthy. In addition, it has become very clear that if your digestion is unhealthy your mouth will be out of balance, and your teeth may become sensitive or weak.

For digestive health, you need a balanced diet, functioning digestive enzymes, and healthy digestive bacteria to turn the food you eat into elements and nutrients that can be absorbed to provide you with the support your body needs. Perhaps the hardest part is to determine the parameters of a balanced diet for ultimate health. My personal advice is to become educated by people who have been successful and who are well informed, and do not let the task be about deprivation or limitations. The truth is that a good diet may simply be to eat real food in moderation with a goal of at least 80 percent of your food plate being a variety of plant foods and vegetables. Once you experience noticeable improvements, it will be easier to be excited about selecting foods for health.

The most noticeable improvements in people's mouth health usually occur when they improve the health of the two most distant parts of their digestive tract—the mouth and the colon—at the same time. Once the health of these locations has been adjusted, it seems improvements will continue along the remaining portions of their digestive tract in a relatively natural sequence. As the digestive health improves, this may even affect the general health of other areas of the body. For example, someone may experience fewer migraines or headaches, reduced allergies, or less fatigue or joint pain.

As we learned in chapter 3, there are over nine hundred kinds of healthy bacteria found in the mouth, and many of them have important functions. Some of these bacteria, for example, help produce nitric oxide from nitrates in saliva. Nitrates are absorbed from certain things we eat, especially many vegetables and fruits, like celery, lettuce, spinach, strawberries, and beets. The nitrates circulate in the blood and are absorbed into the saliva, which takes them into the mouth, where they are processed by healthy bacteria to create nitric oxide, which has many health benefits. Nitric oxide can enhance breathing and blood flow to the brain and heart, but it also has a mouth-health bonus, as it helps control periodontal pathogens and assists in the development of healthy gums around teeth.

To support all the healthy bacteria in the mouth, we must control acidity. This is one of the main reasons I suggest the journey to oral health begins by consuming a tiny amount of xylitol (a one gram piece of gum or a couple of pure xylitol mints) after every meal, snack, or drink. Xylitol works in a number of ways to improve oral health as it can help control mouth acidity, but it also provides fiber to support healthy digestive bacteria, and it breaks down to form butyrate in the colon, which can improve the health of this part of the digestive tract. Xylitol is hygroscopic, which means that it pulls liquids to itself. This means that when you eat a xylitol mint or piece of pure xylitol gum it will stimulate a flow of natural saliva into your mouth. Healthy saliva nurtures probiotic mouth bacteria and helps to mineralize teeth. The quality of our saliva is affected by the following influences:

- Absorption of minerals from the digestive tract (minerals are carried in blood to saliva, where it is available to mineralize teeth)
- Adequate hydration (water is absorbed from our digestive tract and filters into our bodily fluids, and some will become salivary liquids)
- Adequate nutrient absorption from the digestive tract (nutrients support the cells that heal and rebuild tissues everywhere in the body, including our teeth and gums)
- Colon health (influences the absorption of minerals and nutrients and the health of our immune system, which provides antibodies and cells to fight infection—everywhere in the body)

As you can see from this list, digestive health has an incredible impact on mouth health by providing nutrients and hydration for saliva, support for the healing mechanism that can repair damaged teeth and gums, and the nutrients required to support your body's defense system that will help fight infection to allow healing to occur. If your teeth and gums are not healing, it is possible you are not absorbing adequate nutrients, or you may have insufficient blood flow to your mouth. Stress can speed up digestion and leave inadequate time for food to be properly processed or for absorption of nutrients into the blood. Hormones can also affect the health of intestinal bacteria and the digestive process. High-carbohydrate diets and artificial sweeteners (especially Splenda) can affect your digestive pH, and upset intestinal health and your body's ability to absorb nutrients and heal. This is often an undiagnosed problem that can negatively affect the oral and bodily health of someone who is eating a healthy diet yet does not seem to be reaping its benefits.

Throughout life, everything we eat or drink will affect our health and our teeth to some degree. Frequent consumption of sugary foods promotes the conditions that can harm your body and your teeth, and mineral-rich foods have the opposite effect. The outcome for health is what we do regularly, so it really means looking at our normal habits and deciding if they support our health or not. This is also the same process when you have dental problems. You must review your daily habits and decide if they cause more damage than repair each day. If your teeth are sensitive or damaged, then the amount of demineralization your teeth are experiencing outweighs the support that your saliva is providing them for mineralization and repair. The solution is to tip the balance in favor of health by ensuring your habits and diet promote health and that you give your teeth adequate time to interact with undiluted, mineral-rich saliva—an idea we will explore in the next chapter.

CHAPTER 5

Remineralization: Reversing Cavities

Many medical facts are not facts in any sense of the word, they have simply been made up. And that, ladies and gentlemen, is a fact.

—Dr. Malcolm Kendrick, *Doctoring Data*

How do we determine mouth health? We cannot be satisfied with great-looking teeth or believe that the number of fillings we have are an indicator, because these are not true measurements of mouth health. We cannot even celebrate comments by our dentist, because even this can be misplaced confidence. How does your dentist judge mouth health without using some sort of quantifying and health-measuring tool? As you learned in the preface, a group of doctors, dentists, and other health professionals had their own oral health tested at the 2015 Oral Systemic Health Challenge, and the results showed problematic levels of gum-disease bacteria, plaque in their arteries, and even systemic chronic inflammatory markers in their blood. These are dentists and hygienists who relied on meticulous brushing, flossing, and regular dental cleanings to maintain their mouths. They thought that their mouths were healthy, which indicates how impossible it is to determine oral health, or know if harmful pathogens are multiplying in your gums, or know if plaque is building in your carotid arteries. We need a better way to measure invisible mouth health, so we can know if our mouth is healthy or not. Without some clarity, we can imagine that we have a healthy mouth, but if we look through the wrong lens, we may be ignoring problems that are dangerous if left unchecked. We need to know if we are in a situation where small changes and a different approach could help us enjoy a lifetime of less dental treatment and possibly improved general health.

Dental offices normally follow a standard protocol that has been accepted for about four decades, and the routine kicks into gear as soon as you walk through the office door. First, you have a dental cleaning, and then one of the staff will gather data about your teeth and gums by probing with a metal spike to measure pockets in your gums or sticky spots on teeth. X-rays are usually taken, and a camera may magnify your mouth to illustrate cracks in surfaces or other problems so that your dentist can use this information to draw a conclusion about the treatment he or she will recommend for you.

REACTIVE VERSUS PREVENTIVE CARE

Traditional dentistry is based on a find-and-fill approach, and it represents *reactive* dental care. The dentist is looking for damage that can be fixed. You as a patient are rarely involved in this evaluation, and the problem is that there is a high probability that many of these traditional measurements can be false positives or ignore impending problems that at this stage could be reversed easily with effective home care. A *preventive* approach would be a dental evaluation that anticipates your future problems and alerts you to them before you need treatment. This type of care would offer advice about how to make changes for an outcome that would help you *avoid* treatments now, but it would also potentially offer even greater benefits in later life, when repairs of old fillings often become complex and expensive.

Ideally, patients must be involved in preventive care as they need to understand *why* they have dental problems and *how* they can improve their mouth health. Only motivated patients can be enrolled in such a program and make the changes that will reverse their problems. On the other hand, few patients really understand how precious mouth health is and how it connects with overall bodily health. A conversation about the impact of periodontal pathogens on your risk for stroke, for example, could be far more motivating than the silly and inaccurate joke that you should "floss the teeth you want to keep."

The problem is that most insurance systems do not pay for in-depth oral-systemic education at this time. Even the so-called preventive measures that are currently endorsed by the ADA are in fact types of treatment, such as the application of fluoride, sealants, or regular cleanings. We can argue that these things can be helpful for some patients, but none of them address the underlying imbalance in the mouth's ecology, which is the reason for most dental damage. When patients work to improve their mouth health, they will need some kind of reevaluation of their progress, but in most offices, there is no way to monitor if teeth are getting stronger. Most dentists know that oral health affects bodily health, yet there is little financial incentive to promote this fact. Very few dentists are trained to take the salivary tests that show levels of periodontal pathogens—the carotid intima-media thickness scans that show plaque deposits in the carotid arteries—or take A1c or C-reactive protein blood tests to show signs of inflammation in your blood that can alert you to an increased risk for stroke, cardiovascular disease, and other health- and even life-threatening conditions.

SALIVA—OUR NATURAL ALLY

The biggest misconception, in my opinion, is that food causes teeth to decay. If food is the core problem and cavities happened when food becomes lodged in teeth, it would be simple to advise everyone to brush and floss, and this meticulous care would indeed keep everyone's teeth healthy. Certainly there's an element of truth in this food idea, but mouth problems are more complex and must be looked at from a different perspective. Although our dietary selection contributes to mouth health, it is not the actual *pieces* of food, but rather food particles *dissolved* in saliva that flow around our mouth that affect our mouth ecology in a positive or negative way.

This means that rather than food being the enemy, it is liquids and liquid products from food dissolution that influence mouth health, from sugars dissolved in saliva to the acidity of sugarless drinks and sometimes even plain water. Everything we introduce into our mouth can directly affect mouth health in either a positive or negative way. Sugars and carbohydrates create sugary liquids that feed the kind of plaque bacteria that produce acids. Aggressive anaerobic plaque bacteria, which are specifically found in highly infected plaque, can even ferment dairy products and produce very strong acids that easily initiate cavities and trigger a destructive chain of gum problems. Proteins and fats are generally pH neutral, and some may help with mineralization of teeth and promote healthy biofilm.

When you see the various ways that foods have the potential to create dental problems, you understand why trying to limit sweets or control decay though diet alone is an impossible task. If you want to control cavities, it is far easier to embrace your mouth's best ally, which is natural saliva at a nonacidic pH of around 7.4, which is normally found alongside healthy oral biofilm, especially when your diet is low in sugar and carbohydrates and high in mineral-rich, plant-based foods. Check your eating patterns to control acidity, and allocate adequate time each day for your saliva to directly contact your teeth and gums so it can transfer minerals into enamel, where they will build tooth strength and repair any acidic damage.

The production of saliva is a complicated process, and alterations in your general health, nutrition, and hydration will affect its quality and pH. Stress, inactivity, pregnancy, depression, hormones, and medications can create acidic saliva that may be too thin or thick to support mouth health. Poor-quality saliva will have a direct impact on teeth and on the mouth's ecology, weakening teeth and allowing your gums to deteriorate. Saliva flows from three glands on each side of the face, one located in the cheek and two under the lower jawbone.

In addition to liquid from these glands, a component called *crevicular fluid* oozes from around teeth, and there is also input from smaller glands in the mouth, producing a total of about a liter of saliva daily. Saliva is mostly water, but a vital 1 percent is composed of proteins and electrolytes. Healthy saliva aids in digestion, lubricates the mouth, and provides the matrix for healthy biofilm, which can prevent food from sticking between and around teeth. Saliva moistens the mouth to make talking, swallowing, and eating more comfortable, and it helps wash away food particles. If saliva is sufficiently alkaline, it can neutralize acids that could otherwise cause tooth damage, as it is a solution supersaturated with calcium and phosphate ions, the two most important minerals for building and repairing teeth. It's important to know that our saliva has not yet been outperformed by any of the expensive new and heavily marketed mineralizing rinses and pastes. Use your own healthy saliva as an ideal ally for improving your oral health, and work to support its flow and mineral content, and give it adequate time to interact with your teeth and gums to keep them healthy.

The flow rate of saliva varies from hour to hour and from person to person, and its mineral and protein content is influenced by stress, hormonal balance, blood flow, diet, posture, and digestive health. In a healthy mouth, saliva is stimulated as we look at food, a reaction generated by our nervous system. Studies on saliva by J. Ekstrom et al. looked at how the elements in this secretion, especially the enzymes, become modified to fit specific and changing digestive needs as we view and think about the food we are going to eat. As we chew, muscles around our mouth squeeze saliva from the parotid glands that are located in each of our cheeks, and they activate the submandibular and sublingual glands, which are underneath our lower jaw and tongue.

Someone with copious amounts of mineral-rich, protein-rich, and alkaline saliva may manage to achieve oral health with apparent ease. On the other hand, anyone with poor saliva flow or who has acidic saliva will need to be especially careful about their choice of toothpaste, their frequency of eating, and their selection of foods and drinks. Problems begin when teeth do not have sufficient contact with saliva. This can occur if you have frequent snacking or sipping habits or wear braces or a night guard that may prop open your mouth and allow it to become dry. Similar problems occur if your teeth naturally protrude outside the cover of your lips, or if you have lips that do not close over your teeth. This anatomy puts your teeth outside the area of salivary flow, and so they easily become dry, demineralized, and prone to cavities. Your skeletal structure is of course hereditary, and if your entire family has this kind of lip structure, called *incomplete lip closure*, the resultant dental problems may appear to be genetic. The genetic component that influences your anatomy may increase your risk for decay, but when you understand the real problem is about teeth interacting with saliva, this risk is not insurmountable.

There are various ways to encourage saliva to flow and make teeth healthier. Adopt routines that give teeth time to be in contact with saliva, and if you have protruding teeth or know your teeth become dry, ensure you lick them and work saliva over them as often as possible. Xylitol is probably your best ally if you have acidic or poor-quality saliva or a dry mouth. Eating a pure xylitol mint or piece of gum will stimulate a flow of saliva into your mouth, and this saliva is usually at a perfect pH for mouth health. Good nutrition helps mineralize saliva, but even then, saliva pH is not always under your control. Saliva flow increases at mealtimes and slows when you sleep. Early afternoon is a peak flow time, and the dark hours of night are when teeth are most at risk. This is why it is important to ensure your teeth are adequately protected before you go to sleep at night, and no sugary food particles are left to dissolve during the night, a time when we have sluggish saliva and our teeth are at greater risk.

DEMINERALIZATION AND REMINERALIZATION

Dentists call the process of losing and gaining minerals in tooth enamel *demineralization* and *remineralization*, respectively. Calcium and phosphates mineralize tooth enamel, and both these minerals occur abundantly in saliva. A healthy mouth is protected by a thin biofilm on every surface, including the gums and teeth. The biofilm on teeth attracts vital minerals to leave saliva and land on the tooth's outside enamel.

From here, the minerals diffuse deeper into the tooth and move toward any area of shortage to repair and rebuild enamel that has been weakened by previous acidic attacks. The replacement of minerals into deficient areas should occur as soon as possible after acidic attacks to minimize damage and ensure total, immediate repair. When saliva is alkaline, it's rich in calcium and phosphates, which support this natural process of mineralization, keeping teeth strong and densely mineralized. Rebuilding enamel is a natural process, but it can only occur under the correct conditions when teeth are covered by healthy biofilm and they are given adequate interaction time with mineral-rich saliva.

After an extended period of mineral loss, your saliva may not be able to repair this damage, which will leave the tooth weaker and demineralized. Acidic saliva will not have enough minerals for repair, and if you have acidic saliva, it is especially important to minimize loss of minerals and use strategies to strengthen your teeth. Acid attacks occur everytime we sip acidic drinks like coffee, smoothies, or wine. If we sip at five- or ten-minute intervals, substantial demineralization can occur, because there is inadequate time for any repair between the acidic attacks. The secret for protecting teeth from excessive demineralization is to control snacking and sipping, especially in the afternoon hours when saliva is most healing, and use food pairing to minimize demineralization when you choose to sip or nibble. Pure xylitol gum or mints can also help us limit demineralization damage when they are used at the end of every meal, snack, or drink. The flow of alkaline saliva stimulated by eating xylitol will help wash away acids and provide minerals to help heal demineralized enamel.

Demineralization occurs every time our mouth is acidic. The minerals in teeth dissolve into the acid, and the longer our mouth is acidic, the more damage occurs. When minerals have dissolved, a fragile skeleton of enamel remains, like a honeycomb without the honey. In this situation, any pressure or stress on the tooth can cause the enamel shell to break, forming a hole, or cavity. Despite the huge amount of fear, myth, and insecurity in many people's minds about cavities, there is only one way for a cavity to form: Acids in the mouth (from various sources, including acidic saliva, acidic drinks and foods or acids produced by harmful mouth bacteria) dissolve the minerals from a tooth's surface and reduce its strength until a point is reached where some everyday stress overwhelms the weak enamel, and it breaks.

Weak or soft teeth lack minerals, and this is either a problem with inadequate mineral transfer *into* the tooth or excess transfer of minerals *out of* the tooth. We should always address both issues, correcting any mineral-deposit problem while working to prevent mineral withdrawals as much as possible. When minerals accumulate in the surface layers of teeth, the enamel becomes brighter, stronger, and smoother. Imagine teeth as a bank account: If your teeth have too few minerals, it is like a bank with too little money. If your bank account is devoid of money, you will need to take out less and put in more, right? If teeth are deficient in minerals, you must protect them from mineral loss and create a healthy mouth environment that encourages minerals to deposit into them as frequently as possible.

CAVITIES

You cannot win any game unless you have a clear understanding of the rules and the game's goals. If your goal is to avoid cavities, you need to know the exact definition of a cavity, precisely how and why cavities form, and exactly what you can do to effectively stop or avoid them. A lack of knowledge, inaccurate perspective, or ineffective training will mean you never reach your goal, no matter how much effort you put to the task.

A cavity is simply a hole in a tooth, and as mentioned, it occurs only after the tooth's outer shell has been dissolved by acids, which opens up microscopic passages. If your mouth is infected with cavity bacteria, they will use this demineralized passage to penetrate inside the tooth. Corrosive acids are produced by aggressive plaque bacteria, and these are the acids most often responsible for breaching a tooth's surface. Obviously, the stronger your enamel, the better it will resist acid attacks. This is why effective cavity control should always include strategies to strengthen tooth enamel. When harmful microbes burrow inside enamel, they create additional acids that cause deeper demineralization, and this allows them to penetrate further inside the tooth. These bacteria will survive and thrive if they continue to derive energy from their usual food source— sugars from the foods you eat that are dissolved in mouth liquids.

Saliva flows all around teeth like an ocean washing over a coral reef. When harmful bacteria get inside a tooth, they continue to have direct contact with saliva, as mouth liquids are able to travel along the demineralized access passages, opened up as the cavity-forming bacteria gained entry to the tooth. These channels function like a straw and allow these bacteria to feed happily on sugars from any foods or drinks you consume.

The soft mix of cavity-forming bacteria and damaged tooth debris creates a discolored defect known as *dental caries*, or tooth decay, which may look like an inert clay-type substance, but it is alive with bacteria. Dental caries is one of the most prevalent childhood conditions, and repairing teeth damaged by caries is the reason so many children have treatments in dental offices and often require sedation or even a general anesthetic in a hospital setting to fix the damage this disease can cause. As the bacteria continue to multiply, this area of dental caries expands under the tooth's surface, weakening the tooth structure until the enamel covering the area finally collapses. This moment is the time when dental caries usually becomes clinically visible as a hole, noticeable in the tooth's surface and full of brownish decay.

Dental caries is a slowly progressing bacterial infection and a cavity is the eventual defect that is created by this disease. Caries does not happen by chance, is never at a random location on a tooth, and cannot be caused by foods alone, since even sugary foods require processing by cavity-producing bacteria. When cavity-forming bacteria are present in plaque or in a cavity, they will also be floating in saliva, traveling all over the mouth, being transported everywhere saliva goes, and landing on other vulnerable teeth, where the bacteria will launch a similar attack and possibly form similar cavities.

Teeth have different shapes, and some of these shapes make them more vulnerable to the attacks of cavity-forming bacteria. This is why dentists understand the sequence in which teeth are usually damaged. For example, the grooves of molar teeth are more vulnerable than the thick, smooth enamel of a canine or front tooth, and the smooth sides of teeth are more resistant than their biting surface. Because the grooves of molar teeth are generally the most vulnerable locations for decay, seeing healthy grooves is usually an excellent indicator that the rest of the mouth will be healthy, too. There are exceptions, especially for dry front teeth or when people have habits like sucking candies or acidic fruit, which can demineralize teeth in odd areas that are not normally at risk.

One of the most misunderstood messages about teeth involves why cavities form. Patients somehow think that filling this hole or cavity will stop tooth decay, and they do not understand that the same bacteria will continue to damage other teeth, no matter how many have been filled. Conversely, if the disease is controlled with an effective strategy, the actual filling of the cavity becomes less important. We can think of this in the same way as we would view extinguishing a fire, and we all know this is far more important and urgent than fixing the damage it has caused. In a healthy mouth, fillings are only necessary for the structural repair of a defect that is unable to naturally repair and rebuild itself. A filling is not, as many think, a way to stop the mouth's infection, and fillings do nothing to change the imbalance in the mouth's ecology—which is the real, underlying problem.

Something else you should know: Fluoride cannot change or improve the bacterial ecology in your mouth or remove cavity-forming bacteria. Fluoride's only power is that correct use of certain fluoride products can strengthen teeth to resist acidic attack, and it can also help speed the rate of remineralization to help repair any weak or damaged teeth. Complete reversal of a cavity will occur only if the "cavity infection" can be eliminated, which is why fluoride products are unable to reverse or heal cavities when they are used alone. This is vital knowledge as it explains why fluoride is only useful in a limited way and as part of a more complete strategy.

Reversing Cavities

The reason that I wrote my first book, *Kiss Your Dentist Goodbye*, was because I noticed few people in the United States knew that cavities could naturally heal and repair themselves. I wanted to explain how the process of acidic demineralization creates cavities and how reversal is easily possible under correct mouth conditions. Many people in Europe, Australia, New Zealand, Asia, and Japan have known about tooth remineralization for decades.

How much better would it be to use proactive prevention and rebalance an infected mouth ecosystem and establish a protective biofilm before damage occurs? I see dentistry's current reactive approach as similar to playing a whack-a-mole game. This game is one where kids make a frantic attempt to stop little moles from popping out of holes in a table; as one is whacked, another pops up. Filling cavities without concern for the underlying whole-mouth bacterial infection paints a similar picture, whereas a proactive approach would be to remove the moles from this game (i.e., bacteria) and end the "fun" of whacking at them every time they reemerge.

Remineralization is the rebuilding of teeth, and it is a natural process that occurs constantly in a healthy mouth as saliva contacts tooth enamel. This process is slow, but it provides the ongoing repair that helps ensure our teeth remain strong. Tooth rebuilding and breakdown is like the constant breakdown and repair of bones in our body. This ongoing rebuilding ensures that our bones and teeth are restored with new, fresh minerals, allowing them to remain strong and healthy. The good news is that remineralization can be accelerated by a tiny amount of sodium fluoride applied topically to the tooth surface, and this is why I often recommend using a well-formulated sodium fluoride toothpaste or mouth rinse.

Remineralization is the body's way of repairing a damaged tooth, and it is impossible to say at what point the damage becomes too severe for natural repair, especially when correct sodium fluoride products are paired with xylitol, since they work synergistically. Many times, I have helped patients return their teeth to total health, but success is easier to predict if we begin remineralization before the tooth's enamel skeleton has been physically broken. Most small cavities take at least a year to form, and the reversal and repair can happen in a fraction of this time—often in less than three months. In 2008, a group of Australian researchers looked at how easily small cavities can be reversed, and they concluded it may not be ethical for dentists to fill early cavities, because doing so ignores their potential to remineralize. The most important fact is that remineralization will only occur when saliva has the time to interact with teeth and when the biofilm of the mouth is healthy.

Sometimes dentists express concern about trying to reverse a cavity, because they worry about cavity-forming bacteria being too deep inside a tooth. This may have been their teaching in dental school, and without a comprehensive strategy to deal with the cavity infection, I would agree. The caveat is that reversing deep decay requires three methods be used in synergy to address various parts of the cavity problem equation:

1. Change and improve the bacterial ecology in the mouth with frequent use of at least 3–10 grams of xylitol daily.

2. Use my Complete Mouth Care System, which we will explore in chapter 9, to address the dental caries infection inside a tooth without damaging good bacteria or the proteins of healthy biofilm.

3. Use my diet and lifestyle suggestions to improve saliva health and give your teeth time to interact directly with saliva for a few hours every afternoon.

When these strategies are followed, they can be so successful that even caries deep in dentin will reverse. Always remember, the fight is between you and living bacteria inside the carious lesion lodged inside your tooth. These bacteria sit at the end of a straw-like tube, surviving because they continue to derive nutrients taken from *your* mouth, especially any sugars dissolved in mouth liquids. The more often you feed these aggressive anaerobic bacteria with sugars, milk products, or acids, the more destructive they will be. Many people are amazed to think that their own diet is literally feeding the cavity bacteria and keeping them alive in their little cave under the tooth's surface, *every time* they eat or drink supportive products. On the other hand, frequent exposure to xylitol will have the opposite effect and can help limit the propagation of these cavity-forming bacteria. This is why frequent exposure to small amounts of xylitol is so beneficial. There isn't a wound anywhere in the body that can heal until the infection has been stopped. The same principle applies to teeth. The carious area cannot begin to heal and remineralize completely until all these cavity-forming bacteria are controlled.

Cavity bacteria thrive in the acidic conditions that are generated by acidic drinks, juices, lemonades, sodas, fresh fruits, dehydrated fruits, crackers, cookies, sweet treats of all kinds, ice creams, breads, and carbohydrates in every form, as carbohydrates break down to form sugar. This list also includes foods that are organic, gluten-free, or certified healthy. The more frequently we snack, eat, or drink, the quicker cavity bacteria grow, and the more aggressive they become. To eat for a healthy mouth:

- Consider increasing time between meals and snacks.
- Consume sugary or acidic foods and drinks at mealtimes, incorporating them in the meal, and end with 100 percent xylitol to protect teeth.
- End meals or snack between meals with a protein or tooth-safe food (e.g., cheese, chicken strips, turkey, sausage, unsweetened plain kefir or yogurt, celery, avocado, salad lettuce, salty nuts) or xylitol mints or gum.
- Try not to sip constantly, even water (which dilutes saliva). Give

you teeth uninterrupted time to interact with saliva, especially after lunch, when your saliva is healthiest.

Alkaline foods help negate acidity and the damage caused by acidic conditions that occur at the end of almost every meal. Tooth-safe foods are the best snacks between meals, as they do not promote cavities. Making smart food choices will make a big difference in mouth health, especially for children or adults trying to develop and establish a new mouth ecology and end any ongoing problems of cavities or gum disease.

WHITENING TEETH

Teeth that are fully mineralized will be strong, resist damage, and reflect light from their hard, diamond-like surfaces to appear shiny and bright. Healthy enamel will be hard enough to resist staining. Strong enamel that is covered by healthy biofilm will not stain or soak up colors from liquids, like tea or wine. They will be unable to penetrate the tooth surface and stain the tooth. Acid-damaged or artificially whitened teeth are often very porous, and far more likely to stain. Weak enamel is less mineralized, which makes it appear to have a chalky, dull whiteness. This whiteness is not a good sign, and the coloration occurs when light is not reflected normally from the tooth's surface. Although soft enamel may begin by looking white, it will gradually darken and become more yellow. Weak teeth are more likely to break, chip, and crumble. Staining from tea or other drinks only happens if tannins or colored ingredients are able to soak into the porous structure of weak enamel. This is why teeth that have been artificially whitened are at greater risk for staining, and patients are usually told to avoid colored drinks for hours or days after the treatment. Hard, fully mineralized teeth are not at risk for staining.

When you sip wine, tea, or coffee over many hours, the initial damage is the loss of minerals as the acidic drink demineralizes teeth and opens up pores in the enamel surface. This allows the staining to occur, when tannins or colors from the beverage are able to soak into the porous enamel and leave stains on your teeth. The most important protection against this kind of staining is to strengthen your teeth to their maximum state of mineralization. Strong teeth resist staining. Another helpful suggestion is to drink any dark or acidic drinks as part of a meal and end the meal with xylitol.

No matter our intentions, sometimes we may end up sipping acidic drinks, maybe at parties or social events. In these situations, try to interrupt the sips of acidity by nibbling something that is alkaline or tooth-friendly. This is a trick that can also be used for toddlers who have a habit of sipping juices. Between sips, nibble foods that are salty or acid-neutral, like nuts, cheese, cucumber, celery, or some pure xylitol mints or gum.

The more whitening you do, the more likely your teeth will be porous, damaged, and prone to staining. This is because whitening treatments strip teeth of the waxy biofilm protection that normally defends healthy enamel from staining, and the chemicals in most tooth-whitening products also alter the protein structure inside teeth, leaving them less able to resist damage from cavity bacteria. The abrasives and corrosives in whitening pastes and whitening strips etch and scratch teeth to make them appear whiter, but this is a superficial illusion achieved in the same way acids and sandpaper can etch or whiten glass.

Whitening with peroxide occurs as a hydroxyl free radical is released to bleach the deeper layers of teeth, and this can alter the tooth's internal protein structure. Whitening may cause sensitivity to your teeth and damage your gums—damage that may last a few weeks or possibly for the rest of your life. Some people have whitened their teeth and so damaged their gums that it opened up a space that was previously filled by gum tissue, but now this area appears as an empty, black triangle between teeth. Peroxide has also been shown to cause the release of mercury from silver amalgam fillings, which would raise your risk of toxicity from any silver fillings in your teeth (mercury toxicity is believed to cause damage to our body and brain). Recent research corroborates the warnings that have been given in scientific literature for years, even before whitening products emerged into the marketplace in the 1980s. Studies show that bleaching upsets a tooth's live internal tissues in the pulp area and can cause inflammation and damage to these cells in the center of the tooth. In most cases, the damage from bleaching is not apparent immediately, and it may be years before tooth death, enamel weakness, dentin permeability, or changes in the pulp cells are noticed, which can make it difficult for us to link this damage with the whitening and bleaching procedures. Bleaching and the use of peroxide may also roughen tooth surfaces, strip away healthy biofilm protection (leaving the mouth more prone to ulcers), and allow foods to stick to tooth surfaces and lodge between teeth.

Tooth whitening makes no sense to me when I consider it from a health perspective, yet it is a booming business even among avid health seekers, and sales of whitening products in stores and dental offices doubled between 2000 and 2006. There were many studies that have questioned the safety of bleaching, but in recent years, these have become difficult to access. One review by Professor Alberto Consolaro was published in 2013 in the *Dental Press Journal of Orthodontics*, giving clear warnings about the use of peroxide. Even so, most dentists and doctors debate the quality of these studies, and many completely ignore the warnings. The cost of a one-time whitening treatment may be $300 or less, and sometimes this can be offered as a free service. The problem is that a free treatment may cause gum and enamel damage that can create substantial expense in the future, maybe many years ahead. Repeat bleaching is often done annually, and the potential damage that whitening could cause to fillings, enamel, and gums may require dental work of various kinds, including veneers and crowns, cosmetic gum grafting and surgeries, treatment for sensitivity and soft enamel, and even root canals or implants that need special maintenance and bite guards. All this damage could add up over the next few decades, creating the need for treatments and repairs that could potentially total over $50,000 in expenses. Remember, this damage may have been initiated by a *free* whitening treatment. In chapter 9, I will share a safe and natural way to improve your enamel strength with a program that is designed to guard your mouth health and provide healthy teeth that are naturally whiter, shinier, and brighter.

WEAK ENAMEL

Weakened enamel is not able to adequately protect the vulnerable live tissues of the dentin and pulp inside a tooth. If you have damaged or softened enamel, you will usually notice that your teeth feel sensitive to hot or cold temperatures, and this progressively worsens if your teeth continue to be harmed. Eventually, the demineralization damage will become irreversible and potentially result in the death of the tooth. When a tooth has died, the dead part will need to be cleaned and the space blocked with a root filling. Finally, after a root has been filled, the tooth will need some kind of protective covering to prevent the tooth from splitting or absorbing mouth liquids into its core. Most often this means making a gold or porcelain crown. Weak enamel was the cause of this drastic and expensive scenario, yet strengthening enamel is relatively easy and should be something you do daily to prevent these problems.

Under high-power magnification, the design of natural enamel that creates the crown covering of a tooth is seen as an awesome construction. The structure resembles intersecting cathedral arches, radiating in every direction. Small rod-shaped prisms build this arch structure, and the rods are arranged in a pattern that gives healthy enamel incredible resistance to biting forces. The enamel covering a pristine tooth protects the underlying tooth during biting and chewing to resist damage and not harm the opposing teeth. The rod prisms radiate like sunrays or porcupine spines at right angles to the tooth's surface. These rods are longest where enamel is thickest, at the pointy cusps that dig into food as we bite.

Enamel gets progressively thinner on the sides of a tooth, thinning toward the gumline, and it eventually disappears at the junction where the tooth root is covered in cement. As enamel thins, the rod-shaped prisms become shorter, more fragile, and more easily dislodged. Mouth acidity can weaken short rod prisms and loosen them. Damaged enamel crystals may split away from the tooth surface in flakes, leaving a void on the side of the tooth close to the root, at the gumline. When enamel crystals flake at the same time from multiple teeth, a sensitive channel can develop at the gumline. Mouth acidity attacks everywhere, but its damage is first seen on the most fragile crystals, the shortest ones. When these crystals break away, usually simultaneously, a groove will form, and sometimes patients can be blamed for aggressive toothbrushing or tooth grinding.

The underlying problems, however, are loss of the protective biofilm and mouth acidity. I always work with clients to try and determine the reason for these problems and figure out what may have damaged their mouth's ecology and caused acidic damage, so we can ensure their teeth are protected in the future. Sometimes this damage was from acidic saliva that was a consequence of stress, pregnancy, or hormonal imbalance. A dry mouth can make acidic damage worse, and brushing acid-softened teeth after meals or after drinking something acidic like wine can also create serious problems. Whatever the cause, it's important to control acidic damage, and xylitol can be a helpful tool. My Complete Mouth Care System will also help remineralize and hydrate enamel to prevent tooth crystals from flaking away at the sides of your teeth. This protection will help minimize your risk of acidic damage, so we can enjoy wine without dental problems!

When enamel is healthy, it functions as a perfectly engineered helmet that can absorb the strong pressing forces that occur as we bite, chew, or clench our teeth. The average biting force is 160–265 pounds, and a healthy tooth can safely transmit these forces and dissipate them through its structure, so there is no damage to the internal parts of the tooth, the surrounding gum, or the underlying jawbone. When a pristine tooth structure has been cut with a dental drill, even for a tiny filling, this natural mechanism for dissipating forces is compromised, and the tooth will never again function in the natural way. The forces will now be transmitted through the filling until they hit the base of the filling, where they will shoot sideways across the tooth. These unnatural forces often cause microscopic cracks in the enamel at the sides of the tooth and at the widest part, the place where teeth touch adjacent ones, which is an area known as the *contact point*. Cracks in enamel allow mouth liquids and bacteria to enter into the teeth and potentially start cavities at these contact points, tucked between teeth, in places called the *interproximal areas*. Decay at the contact point between two teeth is called *interproximal caries*.

If harmful bacteria live in your mouth, cracks will always be a danger, since they offer a preformed entrance for cavity bacteria to enter and damage your teeth. This is why cavities can easily occur in teeth that have pre-existing fillings, which may have caused stress cracks. Because biting forces are transmitted through all molar teeth with every bite, these cracks can often damage many teeth at the same time. This is why it is not unusual for someone to discover twelve or fifteen *interproximal carious lesions* simultaneously, especially during their teen or young adult years.

Teeth with interproximal caries usually have a history of being cut during sealant preparations or a filling a few years before, something that may have seemed insignificant at the time. The news of fifteen fillings can be shocking, and it should jolt you into action, especially if you understand what this means for the future of your teeth. These lesions are usually quite reversible if you take rapid action, and certainly this would be my recommendation. You must be motivated and do everything possible to balance acidity in your mouth and develop a healthy ecosystem.

It is also important to realize that, from now on, biting forces will always be a danger, since a molar tooth that has been cut will never again have the strength of a pristine, uncut tooth. There is no way to remove this risk, so enamel cracks will always be a concern if you have had sealants or fillings in molar teeth. You cannot change the biomechanics of teeth, but you can reverse an early cavity and restore a tooth to its original pristine form and strength. Remember, this is why it is worth reversing a cavity and avoiding even a small filling. Your teeth are like beautiful diamonds, far too valuable to be drilled and filled if treatment can be avoided. Anyone with fillings should be aware of their risk for cracks and embrace the fact that my system of care will help remineralize cracks every day.

WHITE SPOTS

As discussed, plaque is a thickened layer of oral biofilm that is infected by harmful, acid-producing, cavity-forming bacteria. These bacteria expand the biofilm and thicken it so that sometimes it can form a mass thick enough to be seen and scraped off your teeth. As the harmful bacteria layer on each other, the ones pushed to the inside, close to the tooth, may begin to run out of oxygen. This environment causes them to adapt to these low-oxygen conditions, and as they become anaerobic, they become more aggressive. Anaerobic plaque produces strong acids that harm your teeth and toxins or poisons that cause gum damage and inflammation.

Three weeks of damage by the acids produced by these anaerobic plaque bacteria can pull sufficient minerals from a tooth's surface to create a weakened patch that is visible as a dull and chalky white area in the enamel. These damaged sections are known as *white spots*, and they are not only whiter in color but also weak. The acids damage the enamel, and when it no longer reflects light from its surface in the normal way, this creates the illusion of the enamel being a whiter color.

Fighting Plaque

Xylitol is a superb tool to control damaging plaque bacteria as it makes them less sticky and more easily washed away by good mouth rinsing. Aguirre-Zero et al. have also shown xylitol as particularly useful in helping to neutralize the mouth's acidity in studies published in the 1990s in various journals, including *Caries Research*. A review by J. M. Tanzer in the *International Dental Journal* concludes that xylitol can control the development of thick, infected plaque. As mentioned, xylitol also works in harmony with dilute sodium fluoride to help remineralize tooth enamel more quickly and completely. My Complete Mouth Care System teams with xylitol to effectively heal white-spot damage within a week or two and returns the tooth to its normal strength naturally.

White spots tell us that the tooth's enamel is weak, and the next stage of weakness is that the tooth crumbles, fractures, or becomes a cavity. Often, brown speckles will be visible in the white patches, and this is an indication of the imminent failure in the tooth's structure. White spots are completely reversible, but success depends on remineralizing and repairing them as early as possible. A dental cleaning can shine over a white-spot area, but it will not replace minerals, control the infection, or reverse the damage. Some dentists will etch the area and fill all the porosities with a smear of plastic. This is a quick fix, but in most cases, the repair will soon stain, and subsequent repairs will become larger and more invasive as the years unfold. Once plastic has been put onto or into a tooth, the enamel can no longer repair itself naturally.

FLUORIDE

Now seems a good time to discuss the important and confusing subject of fluoride. First, let's consider that you have just damaged your enamel by drinking something acidic like a soda, a citrus or cranberry juice, or perhaps some apple cider vinegar. If you have alkaline saliva, your tooth enamel will quickly and naturally rebuild itself over the next hour or so. However, if you have acidic saliva, you are not going to be able to naturally reverse this damage, which could lead you to eventually need root canals, crowns, extractions, or implants.

I never recommend drinking fluoridated water, and I believe that fluoride should only be used as a topical application on the outside surface of a tooth. When sodium fluoride is used appropriately, this can speed the repair of demineralized areas and help reverse dental damage. Decades as a clinician has shown me that patients who are unwilling to apply any fluoride to their teeth often endure super soft enamel and dental deterioration, and can end up needing root canals and crowns. I believe that regular use of a little sodium fluoride could prevent this damage, which is why I view the regular use of a little topical sodium fluoride as insurance against future tooth damage. For example, a good paste may help heal and repair interproximal enamel cracks that often occur in the sides of teeth after the enamel is weakened by a filling.

In a perfect world, nothing would damage our teeth, and we would never age or have acidic or dry mouths. Then, it could be argued that fluoride would be unnecessary. In real life, however, many foods, drinks, medications, stress, and hormonal situations—such as occur during pregnancy—are beyond our control and create mouth conditions that put our teeth at risk and in need of extra help. Fluoride will assist the building of minerals into teeth, so they can be strong enough to resist damage, potentially helping us avoid dental repairs or the exposure to filling materials, which could perhaps be considered greater threats to our health.

Sodium Fluoride

Only when your mouth has a balanced ecosystem and healthy saliva will you be able to naturally remineralize damaged teeth. The first step of any mouth rehabilitation should be to limit acidic damage and realize that saliva is our best tool for mouth remineralization. A toothpaste or rinse that contains a tiny amount of sodium fluoride can create an ionic charge on the outside of teeth to help minerals from saliva adhere to the outside surface of your tooth. The use of topical sodium fluoride has been shown to increase the speed of natural remineralization, especially for new adult teeth that erupt in the mouth around five years of age. Used regularly, a little sodium fluoride can strengthen these teeth and prevent demineralization and damage that is caused by acidity. Without fluoride, someone with acidic saliva or a dry mouth will experience minimal or possibly nonexistent remineralization. Regular use of a low-concentration topical fluoride is completely different from using stronger fluorides.

Dilute sodium fluoride has also been shown to work harmoniously with xylitol. If you have cavities, fluoride rinsing twice daily, combined with the use of xylitol after meals and drinks, can dramatically improve your oral health. This approach can help protect adult molars as they erupt in children around five years old, but younger children with no risk for cavities do not need fluoride products. Sodium fluoride is as useful for seniors and adults as it is for school-age children and teens, since teeth are constantly demineralizing and are in need of help to preserve their strength. I cannot repeat too often that I do not endorse drinking fluoride, and this is why children should be supervised when they are using fluoride toothpaste or rinses. I also encourage everyone to spit several times after using any dental products to ensure good clearance from the mouth; do not eat, drink, or wash your mouth for at least an hour, so that your teeth can derive the maximum benefit from fluoride rinsing.

MOUTH ACIDITY

Minerals are lost from teeth whenever they are in contact with acidity, which occurs in everyone's mouth every day. In a healthy mouth, this damage is almost immediately reversed by the natural process of remineralization. Problems only arise when this process is compromised, or when the amount of mineral loss from acidic damage is too prolonged or too frequent, as this will overwhelm and outpace the natural repair mechanism. Acidity is measured as pH, on a 14-point scale, where the low end indicates extreme acidity (like lemon juice). Mouth health and healthy bacteria flourish at a pH just a little above neutral, from pH 7.0 to pH 7.4. We do not know the point at which a higher pH can be problematic.

Almost everyone's saliva pH becomes more acidic at night, or when we are tired or unwell. No one has a fixed salivary pH for life, and if today you test and find you have a neutral pH, this is not a guarantee it will remain neutral in the middle of the night or for the rest of your life. When saliva is acidic, it can dip to a level as low as pH 5.0, which usually occurs during the forty weeks of pregnancy, during times of hormonal imbalance, and at times of stress or depression. Mouth pH is affected by what you eat and drink, and most drinks are acidic, like carbonated water, lemonade, or soda, and some have an acidity level as low as pH 2.2, which can be very damaging to teeth, regardless of the sugar content. Acid reflux, acidic foods, some vitamin lozenges and powders, and even a number of popular oral care products are acidic and may cause widespread demineralization problems.

Mouth pH can be tested with special litmus paper or a pH meter dipped into saliva that is collected in a spoon or small dish. Your morning saliva can be used as a baseline reading, but remember, saliva pH fluctuates easily with stress, travel, extra hours of work, or mouth breathing.

An Acidic Dry Mouth

The acidity of saliva is important, but the damage from acidity is made worse when anything reduces saliva flow and causes a drier mouth, including:

- Snoring at night, when your saliva may be acidic
- Breathing through an open mouth, because your lips do not close because of braces or orthodontic appliances
- Allergies, nasal, or sinus problems that may block the nose and cause mouth breathing
- Stress or depression that reduces salivary flow
- Many medications, including medications for allergies and sinus conditions, stress and depression, and most heart and diuretic medications that have the side effect of causing a dry mouth
- Hormonal fluctuations, including pregnancy

Sipping drinks of any kind, including water, dilutes saliva and reduces the percentage of minerals available in saliva to protect and mineralize your teeth. Saliva shows a circadian rhythm, and its composition changes during the day and night. Saliva is usually most mineralizing in the early afternoon, especially after eating a healthy, nutrient-rich lunch. This means that sipping water in the afternoon will disrupt this ideal time for saliva to heal your teeth, something especially important for someone with weak, decayed, or sensitive teeth.

Dry Mouth and Chemotherapy

We have talked a lot about acidic damage and how remineralization will only occur in an alkaline environment with healthy saliva. This is why I believe it is important to mention my concerns about baking soda (bicarbonate of soda), which of course can make a mouth very alkaline, as it creates a pH of about pH 9.0 when it is in solution. Baking soda is often recommended after chemotherapy and for people with a dry mouth, or who suffer from acidic saliva. The assumption is that baking soda will be helpful because it is alkaline.

Baking soda is a handy cleaning product, because it is not abrasive and is excellent for dissolving grease and removing molds. In the mouth, however, this ability to dissolve fats and grease appears to damage the beneficial proteins that are the foundation of healthy biofilm that covers teeth and stops sensitivity, enamel erosion, and gum recession—particularly for mouths that are acidic or dry. Baking soda appears to strip this protective protein layer away in some mouths, which leaves teeth and gums more vulnerable to mechanical, thermal, and chemical assault.

Baking soda became popular for dental health in the 1920s, when a mixture of baking soda and peroxide was used in a poultice placed on gums and found to stop an invasive and painful gum disease known as *acute necrotizing ulcerative gingivitis*. This infection was caused by an amoebic gum pathogen that attacked the mouths of soldiers living in the trenches of World War I. The poultice was used to kill these aggressive gum pathogens in the era before antibiotics, and it was found to stop this virtually incurable disease and allow the ulcerated gums to heal. The problem was that patients often experienced severe gum recession following this treatment.

Fifty years later, Dr. Paul Keyes suggested a mixture of baking soda and peroxide as a nonsurgical treatment for periodontal gum disease.

Dr. Keyes's method was successful in stopping the infection, but his work also describes problems from tooth sensitivity and recession following the baking soda treatments. Baking soda may have solved some serious gum problems in the early 1900s, but today it makes sense to use a gentler approach that protects the integrity of the mouth proteins, gum tissues, and healthy biofilm. My Complete Mouth Care System, which we will cover in chapter 9, is recommended for anyone with gum disease, cavities, bad breath, sensitivity, or weak teeth, and I suggest using it as preventative and remedial aid before and after chemotherapy.

Acid-Alkaline Influences

The longer your teeth are bathed in healthy, alkaline saliva, the more minerals they will absorb and the stronger they will become. Conversely, the longer your teeth are in contact with mouth acidity, the more minerals will dissolve from their surface and the weaker they will become. Minerals dissolve from enamel at a speed that increases with the acid's strength, escalating by a factor of ten for every single-unit pH drop. This is why we must be concerned about lengthy exposure to acids and the strength of these acids, especially liquids with a very low pH like soda, cider vinegar, lemon juice, cranberry juice, citrus juices, whitening products, and even some mouth rinses. These things can drop pH to as low as pH 2.0 or 3.0 in your mouth. Teeth can reclaim minerals after acidic damage if they are able to immediately interact with healthy, undiluted saliva at a pH of around pH 7.4 so that minerals from saliva will enter into the tooth's surface and replace any missing minerals.

The suggestion to brush your teeth immediately after a meal may sound logical to some people, but not if you understand that your mouth is almost always acidic after a meal. It can take about an hour for this acidity to dissipate. This is why some dentists tell their patients to wait an hour before brushing. If you brush acid-softened enamel, it will easily be abraded or worn. In my opinion, the best solution is to use xylitol at the end of meals, because it stops acidic damage instantly by stimulating a flow of saliva. This means xylitol not only limits acidic damage, but it also creates a flow of saliva to remineralize teeth. If xylitol is not available, an option would be to have a tooth-protective food like whole milk or cheese or to rinse the mouth with water to wash away the acidity. Any problems from acidity after eating will, of course, escalate if you snack or drink many times a day, especially if you have a dry mouth or acidic saliva.

For decades, there have been people who have believed it is important to alkalize the body for improved general health. The belief is that the more acidic your body, the more disease-prone you become. At death, of course, our bodies become acidic and are quickly overtaken by acid-loving bacteria, which decompose our flesh. Louis Pasteur, the recognized father of the germ theory, is said to have somewhat modified this theory while on his deathbed in 1895, saying that the body's terrain, or landscape, was more important than the bacteria that caused disease. In other words, he recognized that sickness and disease generally occur *only* when we allow our bodies *to become vulnerable* to harmful bacteria. We could possibly argue that vulnerability to disease is related to our bodily pH in some way. This is certainly true for the mouth, where a slightly alkaline environment supports a healthy ecosystem that is primed to protect itself and resist cavities, plaque, and gum problems.

Since 2010, there have been great strides in the field of biology, and this has revolutionized our understanding of the diversity of mouth microbes. An improved understanding of the relationship between oral and general health has simultaneously magnified the importance of this knowledge. We now know that the biology of the mouth is far more complex than formerly imagined and that there is great clinical significance to the innumerable microbes that constitute the biofilm on teeth and elsewhere in the mouth. New understanding means we must revisit some traditional dental protocols, especially if we think mouth microorganisms may be pushed into the blood and could potentially cause a transient bacterial event, called a *bacteremia*. We now know that a bacteremia can play a significant role in the development of atherosclerosis and potentially increase someone's risk for stroke or coronary heart disease. This new vision helps us develop clearer goals for our mouth health, but it also changes the way we should view older dental ideas and some traditional dental therapies.

CHAPTER 6

Brushing, Flossing, and Xylitol

The greatest mistake is to continue to practice a mistake.
—Coach Bobby Bowden

The oral health of almost everyone in the United States deteriorates with age, even those who brush, floss, and have regular dental cleanings. Obviously, our current methods of tooth and gum care may slow the damage, but eventually, in most mouths, disease wins this game. Most of us begin brushing our teeth as children, but we may never have an assessment of the effectiveness of our technique for the rest of our lives. Confusion from mixed messaging and stakeholder advertising makes it difficult to know what works and what does not; plus, we do not have adequate methods to measure mouth health, especially when someone has crowns and cosmetically improved teeth that can camouflage festering gums, hide discolored teeth, and mask the ongoing dental damage in an infected mouth. Dentists obviously don't want patients to feel bad about their smile, so many dental problems are blamed on old teeth or fillings, bad genetics, lack of saliva, an enamel defect, or a theory that somehow gums deteriorate and teeth become weaker with age.

However, don't think you have to accept deterioration; remember, gum disease and cavities are completely preventable with effective strategies. You may be proud of your meticulous brushing habits, but it may be time to take a closer look and see if they are effective enough to defend you from dental and gum problems. In this chapter, we will discuss the importance of brushing and pairing this with preventive oral-care products that really work. We will also explore the many benefits of xylitol and shed some light on how flossing may not be the priority you once thought.

IMPROVING YOUR BRUSHING HABITS

Key nutrients and cells in saliva are the true workhorses that maintain our gums and teeth by providing constant healing and repair. This is why it is so important to give our mouth adequate time to interact with this major contributor to our oral health. Never blame yourself or think you have incurable dental problems. I hear sad stories of people who continue to use an ineffective ultrasoft toothbrush, because it was suggested by their specialist as he or she simultaneously informed them they would need ongoing periodontal treatments for the rest of their lives. Instead of a soft brush, why not try a firmer medium brush and a new system of care? Who knows? Maybe you can surprise your periodontist with improved mouth health at your next visit!

Toothbrushing can be difficult, especially if you have reduced arm movement because of arthritis or a stroke, which can make the essential gum brushing movements difficult. Medical conditions like diabetes or habits such as smoking reduce circulation to the body's extremities, which include the gums, and this is why some patients are at increased risk for gum disease. Cortisol, a body hormone released when we experience stress, also changes the quality of saliva in our mouth and stifles circulation to our gums, which is why stress can be a risk factor for many oral health problems, including bone loss and periodontal disease.

But don't give up! First, buy some new toothbrushes, and ensure they are not too soft. You'll want to concentrate on reaching all the areas of your gums: even higher above, on the inside areas, and below your teeth in the areas of the teeth's roots. A good gum massage will work wonders if it brings healthy nutrients and cells to fight any cavities or gum problems. In some cases, a battery-operated brush can be useful, since the vibrations help to stimulate circulation when dexterity or access to the mouth is difficult. In other situations, when the vibrations are not tolerable, cleaning the gums with a manual brush or even a sponge or cloth may be your best option. The tool you use is not as important as your method and the results you achieve from using it.

Gum massage brings blood and an associated lymphatic flow to help resolve any infection and brings healing nutrients to the teeth and gums. Brushing *teeth* per se has little influence on whether or not you have cavities, especially if you have a mouth teeming with harmful bacteria and are using an infected brush or bad toothpaste. You can brush many times a day and yet continue to experience bad breath, bleeding gums, and dental decay. Conversely, if you have healthy saliva, a good diet, and smart eating patterns, you may decide not to brush as often and still be able to enjoy a cavity-free mouth. I do not suggest you abandon brushing, but it is important to know that brushing is never a guarantee for a cavity-free mouth.

Brushing with an infected toothbrush can transfer harmful bacteria from external sources, such as from people who have flossed above your brush, leaving bacteria that can multiply in its bristles. Brushing with an inaccurate aim can cause erosion in a tooth's surface if your mouth is acidic or if you use abrasive toothpastes. Brushing techniques that target teeth and do not reach your gums will leave plaque at the gum margins in an infected mouth. The fresh-tasting minty paste can create the illusion that your mouth is clean, but don't be fooled. Many toothpastes, including apparently healthy ones, often contain ingredients like glycerin that may inhibit remineralization and products like baking soda or peroxide that can be problems or strip teeth of a healthy biofilm. This is why selecting appropriate products, toothbrushes, and using good gum-massage techniques are important.

A FEW TIPS

There are a few things you can do to improve your daily brushing habits. They include:

- Using a *clean* and *appropriately sized* brush that is not too soft
- Learn *how* to brush with techniques that generate circulation in the gum area to promote tooth and gum health
- Use a *helpful paste* that ideally delivers benefits to teeth and does no harm; dry brushing without any toothpaste is a better option than using a harmful product

Brush Your Gums

Everything would be so much easier if toothbrushing had been called *gum brushing* or *gum massage*. Our toothbrushing description was born in the 1900s when people thought brushing was to remove food from teeth. At this time, no one knew that cavities were caused by a bacterial infection or that toothbrushes could, in fact, be a part of the problem. The idea of brushing and cleanings—and eventually the idea of floss—was to mechanically and meticulously remove particles from every surface around a tooth. The problem with this method is that if your mouth and saliva are infected, this is *inadequate* care. This is why cavities and gum disease are so prevalent today, as this basic technique does not address the bigger whole-mouth problem of an infected oral ecosystem and the bacterial transmission in saliva. Scorched-earth tactics with strong fluoride or antiseptics disable both the bad and good bacteria, and brushing does not correct an imbalance of the mouth's ecology. Effective strategies, on the other hand, must be designed not only to control any infection but must simultaneously nurture healthy bacteria and their associated biofilm if we are to achieve ultimate success and sustainable mouth health.

Our immune system is a powerful ally for improving bodily health. Good circulation throughout the body is vitally important for the health of all our tissues, and our gums are no exception. Blood transports many cells and nutrients, and important immune cells are carried in the lymphatic system, which flows around our body and can remove harmful bacteria. The blood transports minerals and healing nutrients, so tissues can heal themselves after the immune system has cleared and resolved any area of infection. Without an adequate blood flow, neither cleanup nor healing processes can occur, and without assistance, our gums do not normally receive a sufficiently vibrant blood flow.

Hospital personnel are familiar with wounds that never heal, often in the elderly or patients with diabetes or poor circulation. The secret to mouth health lies in stimulating and encouraging blood flow to the areas of the gums and teeth, using a bacterially clean toothbrush and a good brushing technique. Young children and dynamic adults may jump around enough to naturally stimulate gum circulation, but as we slow down (or in the case of injury or disability), our toothbrush may become our mouth's only ally.

Gum tissues are extremely vascular and filled with tiny capillaries, so when we stimulate circulation in this area, the results can be positive and quick. Yoga inversions that lower your head below your heart can also help gum circulation. If anyone suddenly becomes diabetic, sedentary, or confined to a wheelchair or hospital bed, even for just a few days, their risk for developing gum problems, without appropriate care, can increase.

The goal of gum brushing is to actively stimulate circulation around every tooth, front and back, and on the inside and outside of both jaws. This kind of stimulation will bring blood to the roots of your teeth in these areas and also to the surrounding gums. The blood supply will carry cells to fight infection and nutrients for the wound-healing process. This is why a very soft brush will usually be inadequate or even a waste of your time. Soft brushes were originally fashionable in the era when dentists encouraged patients to oscillate the bristles inside tiny gum pockets around teeth to remove food particles.

The toothbrush now has a different purpose in our fight for gum health. Currently, there is no scientific measurement to categorize toothbrushes as to their stiffness, softness, or hardness. Almost all brushes today are labeled soft, and it may be a challenge to find a brush firm enough to help, but it is worth the effort. If your brush is too soft, you may not be aware of how ineffective it is. On the other hand, if your brush feels too hard, you can always soften the bristles under warm water.

With the exception of electric toothbrushes, many brush heads are too big and difficult to maneuver around your mouth. In general, a toothbrush head should be small, and the handle should be comfortable to grasp. You might think that a larger head means more bristles, but access in difficult areas is probably more important, specifically on the upper outside and lower inside areas along your back teeth. For some of my clients, I suggest a brush designed for teens or young adults. Basically, you want a brush that fits your mouth. And brushes with small heads are generally easier, especially if you have crowded teeth.

FLOSSING

The United States sells about five million kilometers of floss per year, and I suggest that few dentists have dared to dispute or reject flossing because of an underlying fear that this appears heretical. When I began to voice flossing concerns years ago, many people were surprised, but they were not aware of the science about how cavities form, and they often believed cavities were random phenomena or were caused by food stuck between teeth. Today, we know that cavities are a biofilm infection and that a healthy mouth depends on nurturing healthy bacteria and healthy saliva in the ways I have discussed in this book.

There are no studies to support flossing as a method of protecting teeth. Anyone with cavities, gum disease, or plaque buildup may have been told to floss more, but I suggest you use caution and begin instead by using xylitol and my Complete Mouth Care System for at least 6–8 weeks before you begin flossing or have a dental cleaning appointment. I suggest this because flossing cannot help you improve your mouth ecology, and there is risk that flossing and cleanings could push bacteria into the blood from your infected mouth. If you have a problem with food being stuck between your teeth, this will gradually resolve as your mouth becomes healthier; in the meantime, small interdental brushes may be useful for extra plaque control in problem areas.

Researchers at the University of Applied Sciences in Amsterdam searched the scientific literature to check the effectiveness of flossing and compared it to brushing. Using meta-analysis, the researchers evaluated the data and showed no benefit of flossing over brushing alone when they measured plaque or gingivitis and that flossing without toothbrushing had no benefit at all. Two of the studies involved dental students—whom, one imagines, should have had an improved knowledge of flossing—yet this group did not show any better outcome than the general population.

During the past thirty years, I have helped thousands of patients and clients improve their oral health, yet I have never once recommended flossing as the answer to oral health problems. Many of us who grew up outside the United States never considered flossing important. Working as a dentist in other countries during the 1970s, I saw patients who enjoyed amazing oral hygiene but who never flossed. Conversely, I have witnessed hundreds of patients in the United States who are paranoid about flossing and carry devices and floss everywhere, yet their oral health remains poor.

There is obviously a debate over the subject of flossing, but we should all agree about the danger of flossing if we have infected, swollen, or inflamed gums. I also believe flossing may cause sensitivity and contribute to gum recession, and I suggest that people with gum recession or sensitive teeth take a two-week (or longer) abstinence from flossing that I call a *flossing holiday*. It is remarkable how this change can improve gum recession and sensitivity. As mentioned, the other concern is the danger of flossing in an unhealthy mouth. This is why, if you are told by your dentist or hygienist that you need to floss more, I suggest you begin with xylitol and my other strategies to improve your mouth health before you begin flossing. You may also want to take a salivary test to find out if you have any periodontal pathogens breeding under your gums. For anyone with a *healthy* mouth who really wants to floss, I suggest the best time for flossing is at the toothpaste stage of my Complete Mouth Care System, because flossing will move a little toothpaste between your teeth into the interproximal areas, where the toothpaste could provide some extra benefit.

Never allow yourself to be blamed for cavities because of a lack of flossing. Dental statistics suggest that 5 percent of patients floss correctly and enjoy healthy mouths, but I believe it is more likely that this population group has naturally balanced mouth chemistry, healthy saliva, and good habits to support mouth health anyway.

—

In 2012, Helen Rumbelow, a reporter for the London *Times*, called me on the phone while searching for an expert on oral health. She was writing an article about flossing and wanted to pick my brain on the subject. It didn't take long for me to explain my heretic thoughts about floss and the complete lack of scientific support for flossing—not at all what she had expected to hear. I gave Helen the details of my Complete Mouth Care System, and she decided to give it a try. Prior to our conversation, she had flossed avidly. Before making the change, she visited her dentist for a report on her mouth health. She was given a six out of ten. Then, Helen asked what her hygienist believed would happen if she gave up flossing. As you can imagine, the description was pure disaster: plaque, calculus, bleeding, and the demise of her mouth.

Helen was a brave reporter who wanted a good story, so she began to use my regimen with interest and a certain degree of fear. Four weeks later, she returned to her dentist's office for review, without telling them about the changes she had made. Her hygienist was amazed by the state of her teeth, which showed dramatic improvement and now had no bleeding spots and no sign of plaque or inflammation. Helen followed up by talking with the chief of the British Oral Health Foundation and the professor emeritus of dental public health at University College, London. Both dentists agreed that xylitol was a wonderful adjunct for oral health and that it could prevent accumulation of plaque. They agreed that dentists should be aware of the power of xylitol but said that dentists get "bogged down" in the mechanics of dentistry. These experts also corroborated that flossing was not supported by science and is almost completely useless. Needless to say, Helen's article ignited a firestorm and created a flurry of questions on both sides of the Atlantic.

I was interviewed by the BBC World Service and discussed flossing with a number of eminent dentists, who all agreed with me, yet they concluded by saying we must continue to support flossing. In the summer of 2016, an article was published in the United States by the Associated Press, commenting again that there is no proof flossing works. The article created a similar volcano of reaction, with the dental associations and periodontal experts unable to accept these findings. One professor even blamed the poor flossing results that had been documented in the studies on patients who did not floss properly.

RINSING TEETH

Rinsing teeth with a well-selected liquid seems to be a far superior adjunct for oral care than floss, and it will usually yield better results than flossing. Rinses will travel all over your mouth, between teeth, and to all the places that mouth liquids travel. This means that mouth rinses can access grooves in teeth, move around difficult areas behind wisdom teeth, and even get into cavities and under crowns if those are problem areas in your mouth.

Rinses can be great for oral health, but not all rinses are the same or equally effective. In fact, they vary dramatically, and some offer benefits for teeth, others, for gums; some are flavored water, and the worst ones can even be very harmful and upset your mouth health even after one rinse. All these good or bad outcomes depend on the specific ingredients, textures, and acidity levels of each rinse. This is why we need to select mouth rinses for a particular purpose and adjust our method of using them to maximize the desired results.

For example, a rinse like chlorine dioxide is very useful, because it will create oxygen in the small spaces where periodontal bacteria live. Oxygen can disrupt the dangerous anaerobic bacteria that cause gum disease but only if we allow adequate time for the rinse to work; otherwise, the benefits will be lost or reduced. It is also necessary to know where you may have problems; if, for example, you have periodontal problems around your lower front teeth, you must tip your head to ensure the rinse has time to bathe this area of your mouth.

The array of rinses available in the United States today is difficult to navigate, and most dentists are overwhelmed by advertising, sponsored studies, and insufficient time to explore these products or document long-term outcomes. Some professionals accept free samples to give away, and this can confuse patients and derail them from an effective to a less effective product.

One shocking fact is that many rinses today are acidic, with a pH low enough to damage root cement and even tooth enamel. The only acidic rinse that is safe for teeth is one containing dilute sodium fluoride, since the benefits of the fluoride are enhanced in a slightly acidic solution. A number of well-advertised and often esteemed non-fluoride and "natural" rinses are as acidic *as a can of soda* with pH scores between pH 4.0 and 3.3. Another shock is that rinses recommended for dry mouth are often sufficiently acidic to pull minerals out of tooth enamel and root surfaces. Acidic rinses are particularly damaging in a dry mouth. I believe everyone should check products they use regularly, possibly using an inexpensive pH-testing meter.

If you have any cavities or gum disease or are at risk for developing them, certain mouth rinses can be helpful, particularly when used in a special sequence, which we will cover in chapter 9. The rinses I suggest work in harmony with each other and also with the toothpaste I recommend. The choice and order of these rinses is exact and important, and the outcome of the routine depends on using the correct products in the correct order to enable harmonious interactions *between* the products.

CLEANING YOUR BRUSH

Toothbrushes need twenty-four hours between uses to dry in open air. Many years ago, I looked at an infected toothbrush under a microscope, and I still remember seeing crawly bacteria on the brush and how they completely disappeared when the brush was cleaned for a few seconds in bleach or Listerine, then rinsed and allowed to dry. After a single use, all the bacteria in the mouth are transferred to a toothbrush. Even the latest designs of toothbrushes are easily infected, and studies show it makes no difference if you use a new brush: The brush becomes infected after one use.

My recommendation would be to store your brushes in a dry, clean area away from the toilet and to consider a rigorous routine for toothbrush cleaning and replacement, particularly if you are fighting gum disease or cavities. Simply swish the bristles of the brush *daily*, preferably in a drop of an undiluted essential oil antibacterial rinse, like Listerine, for a couple of seconds. Rinse the brush under running water and then store it—bristles up, in a cup or holder—so it can air-dry completely for twenty-four hours between uses. Remember that bacteria lodged inside biofilm will die when they dry. This means that in order to brush twice a day you will need, at a minimum, two brushes. I think it is often a good idea to select two brushes that are different designs, to make brushing feel a little different each time you brush.

If your bathroom conditions are damp, mold or bacteria can grow on your brush, especially if you store it under a cover or inside a bag. Storing your brush close to another one could allow transfer of bacteria from one brush to another. Carrying any toothbrush in a plastic case, in the carry compartment of your vehicle, or in a gym bag is a recipe for disaster. UV toothbrush sanitizers may seem a good idea, but even the manufacturers admit they only kill 99 percent of bacteria. From my clinical experience, I worry that this 1 percent they fail to kill may be an aggressive periodontal pathogen, a frightening microbe called *Aggregatibacter actinomycetemcomitans*. This particular pathogen can cause a rapid form of periodontal disease in adolescents and has been implicated in infective endocarditis. It is also the periodontal pathogen identified in atherosclerotic plaque, which can block arteries and cause heart attacks and stroke. The ADA's position on the cleanliness of your toothbrushes is surprisingly nonchalant, which seems strange considering the fact that so many adults in America have gum disease. The ADA does, however, recommend people susceptible to infections should use "a higher level of vigilance."

XYLITOL

In addition to proper brushing and care of your brushes, I believe that xylitol is a key part of any healthy mouth program. This is because xylitol can quickly bring saliva into your mouth, limit acidity, and help control plaque growth. Xylitol also nurtures and supports good mouth bacteria and appears to aid mineral absorption into tooth enamel and the transfer of minerals into deeper parts of a tooth for more complete mineralization. Xylitol also helps make harmful plaque bacteria slippery, so these bacteria are more easily rinsed away during oral care. Finally, by using xylitol as your ally, you can nurture healthy mouth bacteria and develop a healthier and more protective mouth biofilm.

—

For many years I lived and worked as a dentist in Rochester, New York. During this time, I co-owned a restaurant quite famous in the 1980s as one of the first to offer cappuccino coffees. Our restaurant made Swiss cakes and European pastries, and the staff were provided with a constant supply of broken cookies, pieces of cake, and treats to taste, along with coffee and limitless soda from a fountain in the waiters' area. To freshen their breath, the staff consumed breath mints, multiple times a day. Familiar with xylitol from my career in Europe, I asked why they did not eat xylitol mints. When no one had any idea what I was talking about, I decided to start making xylitol peppermints and put them in a dispenser at the back of the restaurant. Every waiter was able to purchase a small handful for a quarter and nibble them over the course of his or her shift. Quite rapidly, the staff noticed improvements in their oral health, and many became so interested that they began using my other mouth care strategies and the rinses and toothpaste I recommend. Now, over twenty years later, many of these individuals stay in touch and let me know how much they enjoy their ongoing oral health success.

Health Benefits

Xylitol is a low-calorie and diabetic-safe sweetener, and it has been central to my strategies for mouth health for a long time. Xylitol is such an amazing product that I was stunned to find that it was virtually unknown in the United States as late as the 1980s. Xylitol was used in Europe over a hundred years ago as a natural diabetic sugar alternative and was used as an intravenous support for diabetic patients during surgery. It was chosen for its safety, its freedom from the insulin pathway, and its ability to keep the blood glucose of diabetic patients stable during stressful surgical procedures. Xylitol was commonly used as table sugar in homes during sugar rationing in Europe during the 1940s, and in the 1960s, it became popular to help cut sugar cravings and as a chewing gum for smoking-cessation programs.

Xylitol can be extracted from the woody fibers of birch trees, but it is also found in numerous vegetables, fruits, corn husks, and even the human body. In its granular form, xylitol looks and tastes like ordinary table sugar but with a slightly fruity overtone. The difference, however, is that xylitol's effects are almost the exact opposite of sugar, so it nurtures the healthy mouth bacteria, makes plaque slippery, and is useful for digestive health. Xylitol should not be classified as either a sugar alcohol or an artificial sweetener, because its structure differs completely from other members of both these groups. Xylitol is a unique five-carbon (or pentose) sugar, and people are amazed how sweet and delicious it tastes. Some people, especially special-needs patients or dementia patients who are physically unable to eat mints or gum, may benefit from consuming xylitol in baked goods, such as puddings and custards;

sprinkled onto foods or used in drinks; or even wiped over their mouths at the end of meals. The only setback to baking with xylitol is that it cannot be caramelized, and because it has antifungal properties, it inactivates yeast.

Xylitol is a prebiotic fiber food that supports mouth and intestinal probiotic bacteria, and in the colon, it digests to form butyrate, which is a compound that helps support and heal the cells of the colon lining. Xylitol does not dissolve in cold water, but it dissolves easily at room temperature, and once dissolved, it will stay dissolved, even when chilled. Adding xylitol to water may be helpful when higher doses of xylitol are used, as they are in Europe for women with osteoporosis. Doctors who believe in xylitol for bone benefits often suggest an amount of up to 20 grams of xylitol daily. Again, if you are diabetic and choose to replace all the sweeteners in your diet with xylitol, my suggestion is to begin slowly, gradually increasing the amount added to your diet (talk with your doctor before you begin). Any form of xylitol will benefit digestive health, although people with unhealthy digestion should begin using xylitol in very small amounts, maybe 1–3 grams per day in small, divided amounts at first. People with digestive imbalances will develop adequate tolerance to xylitol's special hygroscopic effects, but this can take a few months. For people with a leaky gut, xylitol may allow body liquids to flow through the leaky gut lining and into the gut, which can cause loose stools. Anyone with leaky gut should begin slowly, as mentioned, using just one gram of xylitol at the end of one or two meals each day and then gradually adding more as they become tolerant and their digestive health improves.

Regular use of at least 3 grams of xylitol daily will improve the quality of the biofilm that covers your teeth and mouth, although less than this amount on a regular basis may not show these benefits, which is why some people do not see oral health improvements. Improvement in the oral biofilm may positively affect adjacent areas of confluent biofilm, such as areas in the nose, mouth, throat, and possibly the lungs, but if you struggle with nose, sinus, ear, or acid reflux issues, a xylitol nasal spray may be a useful adjunct as you improve your mouth health. For young children, just as xylitol reduces the number of sticky plaque bacteria on their teeth, it also appears to reduce the number of sticky bacteria in their eustachian tubes and reduce the incidence of middle-ear infections. As harmful bacteria disappear, healthier and nonsticky bacteria will take their place, which means that the ecologies of the mouth, nose, and middle ear will often improve together, and you may notice fewer ear, nose, and throat infections.

Recommended Daily Amount of Xylitol for Oral Health

The total quantity of xylitol consumed each day for oral health should be equivalent to 1 and 2 teaspoons of xylitol (1 teaspoon is about 5 grams). This is recommended for children and adults, but studies show that teeth benefit most from tiny, multiple exposures to xylitol each day—ideally 1–2 grams at each exposure to total between 6.5 and 10 total grams per day. This amount, used regularly, can radically change the profile of bacteria in an infected mouth within a year.

Of course, reducing harmful plaque is one goal, but feeding or supporting a healthy mouth ecology is another part of this strategy and works best when regular sugar and carbohydrates are restricted in the diet. Be aware that studies indicate that less than 3 grams of xylitol per day may not provide any oral health benefits and that, as the number of exposures per day increases, so do the clinical benefits. Over 10 grams per day may not give you any additional dental health benefits, and at this amount, oral health changes appear to plateau. Remember that increasing the frequency of xylitol consumption and considering the best timing will be your way to maximize its benefits. I suggest you strive for a 1-gram serving of xylitol (ideally as two 0.5-gram mints or a 1-gram piece of gum) five times each day after meals, snacks, and drinks.

For maximum dental benefit, do not consume your daily xylitol at once—for example, do not put a teaspoon of xylitol in a cup of tea and expect to see results. Xylitol works in the various ways we have discussed, and we can maximize its effect when it is consumed after meals, drinks, and snacks. Mints, gum, and granules work equally well for reducing plaque, although mints and gum are more convenient and an easy way to count up your dosage to an effective level, especially if you are fighting cavities or gum disease. Check the amount of xylitol in the products you select, since the amounts vary, and companies are allowed to round up the amounts on their nutrition labels.

Correct use of xylitol can gradually eliminate plaque and help protect teeth from cavities. In the first five weeks of using xylitol, you may notice cleaner-feeling teeth, but it takes about six months of regular use to fully change your mouth ecosystem and for you to feel the benefits of having healthier bacteria in your saliva and mouth. Infants and toddlers without decay or plaque can benefit from xylitol, and they will develop a healthier mouth ecosystem even with very small amounts. An effective dosage of xylitol for infants and toddlers is between 1 and 3 grams per day (¼ to ½ teaspoon of granular xylitol).

The other thing to remember is that people with delicate digestive health or leaky gut may not tolerate larger amounts of xylitol at first, so be sure to work up slowly, introducing xylitol by using one mint or one piece of gum at the end of meals, two or three times per day, keeping the total amount to around 3 grams per day for the first month. Then, increase the amount gradually over several months until you reach the ideal amount of 6–10 grams per day (which would be 12–20 half-gram mints, or 6–10 pieces of gum).

Xylitol Gum and Candies

In its granular form, xylitol can be used for baking. It also tastes delicious as chewing gum and healthy, tooth-friendly mints and candies. Since the 1960s, it has been given to preschool children in Finland as part of a public oral health measure. Many studies have looked at xylitol's dental health benefits, and a number of impressive studies were conducted in the 1970s by researchers at the University of Michigan.

Making xylitol a regular part of your daily routine is easy, and this is the best way to experience its benefits. You can eat it as candy, chew it as gum, or use it as a breath mint or spray. When you expose your mouth to a tiny amount with regularity, you will create major changes in the biological health of your mouth. Studies show that five or more exposures per day are ideal, and it appears xylitol's benefits are greatest when it can alkalize your mouth at the end of meals or after snacks.

Granular xylitol can be eaten or used as crystals or made into a solution to wipe, rinse, or brush onto the teeth of babies, the elderly, bedridden patients, or simply to avoid commercial toothpastes and rinses. Xylitol used in this way is a good choice if you are simply looking for a harmless tooth cleaning product with no chemicals and providing you

Here is a table that outlines why xylitol is a key part of my strategy for mouth health.

THE HEALTH BENEFITS OF XYLITOL	
Helps Replace Bad Oral Bacteria with Good	**Prevents Plaque and Cavities**

1. Xylitol reduces harmful plaque bacteria, not by killing them, but by making them slippery, so *plaque bacteria are easily rinsed off teeth.*
 	
2. Xylitol feeds and promotes healthy oral bacteria and a healthy oral biofilm to protect teeth and make them:
  i. Less sensitive to hot and cold (thermal protection)
  ii. Less vulnerable to cavity bacteria (bacterial protection)
  iii. Less likely to be abraded or develop grooves at the gumline (mechanical protection)
  iv. Less likely to be demineralized by acid attacks (chemical protection)
	1. Xylitol does not energize the plaque bacteria that comprise infected biofilm, so it helps *reduce infected plaque on teeth.*
	
	2. Xylitol helps reduce acids in an unhealthy oral biofilm, which means teeth will suffer *less acidic damage.*
	
	3. Xylitol helps *create a flow of saliva to help clean teeth and provide minerals for remineralization.* This is very helpful for people with poor salivary flow or dry mouth.
	
	4. Xylitol mints and gum help stimulate saliva flow to *reduce acidic damage after eating or drinking.* If xylitol is consumed three or four times per day after meals, it will eliminate three or four hours of acidic tooth damage, every day.

Prevents Transmission of Bacteria	Heals Cavities and Strengthens Teeth	Benefits Whole-Body Health
1. Xylitol promotes healthy oral bacteria and consequently *helps limit the spread of cavities within circles of family and friends.* Xylitol has been shown to *control the spread of cavity bacteria from mothers to their infants.*	1. Xylitol stimulates a flow of saliva when it is in the form of a mint, gum, or granules. (This effect is not elicited when xylitol is dissolved in water, since this benefit is created by xylitol's hygroscopic effect.) Mineral-rich saliva will *aid mineralization of teeth.* 2. Xylitol works synergistically with dilute 0.05 percent sodium fluoride to maximize the healing that they both offer. Teeth will be *strengthened and mineralized, and early caries will be encouraged to self-repair.*	1. Xylitol may be a good alternative to help *cut sugar cravings.* 2. Xylitol has been shown in high-performance athletes to *prevent catabolic muscle breakdown.* 3. Xylitol is used in European countries for *osteoporosis benefits* 4. Xylitol contributes fiber for digestive health and has *one-third the calories of sugar.* 5. Xylitol offers an alternative for diabetics and people who want *a healthy sugar.* 6. Xylitol is digested to form butyrate in the colon, a short-chain fatty acid that *maintains the health of cells in the colon lining.*

have no need of other ingredients that could offer enamel protection or remineralization help.

However, while xylitol is useful to control plaque and nurture healthy mouth bacteria, xylitol cannot eliminate periodontal pathogens from periodontal gum pockets, and it cannot eradicate immature plaque spores or certain other bacteria found in an infected mouth. This is why xylitol may not give you adequate protection when used by itself, especially if you are experiencing cavities or gum disease.

Xylitol is a great way to limit the damage caused by acidity after meals. Usually teeth are damaged for close to an hour, every time we eat or drink. Xylitol helps generate a flow of saliva, which will wash away acidity and can provide minerals to heal any damaged areas of tooth enamel. This effect is achieved because xylitol is hygroscopic, which means it attracts water to itself. When you consume xylitol as mints or gum, they pull some saliva into your mouth from small salivary glands in the roof of your mouth. In most mouths, this saliva is mineral-rich and alkaline, which is conducive to tooth health and repair.

Remember that this effect cannot occur if xylitol is added to water, because the hygroscopic effect is nullified. Drinking xylitol water can be useful, but it cannot contribute to remineralization and the reversal of cavities in the same way as is achieved by regularly eating some mints or gum. By consuming xylitol regularly, you will encourage natural tooth healing, and the more often you eat xylitol, the more help you will be giving your teeth and gums. Xylitol mints or gum will also help people with dry mouth by creating a flow of saliva, and studies have shown that using xylitol mints daily can reduce the amount of root decay in high-risk patients by 40 percent.

Please note: *Xylitol should not be given to animals*—particularly not dogs. There are many human foods that are dangerous for dogs—grapes, chocolate, and raisins, to name a few. Xylitol is another of these foods, and it's best kept away from animals.

BEWARE: FAKE XYLITOL

Xylitol is expensive and is often mixed with cheap but similar-sounding sweeteners. For example, xylitol is sometimes mixed with sucralose or other artificial sweeteners. Marketing on these packages often advertise the *benefits of xylitol*, and people wrongly believe that xylitol is another artificial sugar or a sugar alcohol similar to sorbitol, maltitol, or mannitol, which are all products well known for giving people stomach cramps, bloating, gas, and acid reflux symptoms. As xylitol emerged in America in the early 2000s, a major gum manufacturer sent large bags of sorbitol gum that contained a tiny amount of xylitol to every dentist in the country, advertising that this gum was "now with xylitol." Dental staff chewed this gum, unaware it was mainly sorbitol. Many were disappointed at the lack of dental benefits, because there was insufficient xylitol. High doses of sorbitol also cause gastric upsets, acid reflux, and bloating, which many people incorrectly attributed to xylitol and not the real culprit, *sorbitol*.

Another sweetener that is less expensive than xylitol is erythritol. Xylitol is often mixed with erythritol to create a cheaper product. Recently Cargill, the largest privately held global corporation in the United States in terms of revenue, became involved in the erythritol supply chain, so you can expect to hear more about erythritol. Erythritol is derived from corn, and because the body does not recognize this product, it will be touted as calorie-free. Like all zero-calorie products, this may not be a healthy attribute, and I do not promote erythritol or suggest you mix it with xylitol or allow yourself to be swayed by research that asks you to believe that erythritol is superior to xylitol.

BAD BREATH

People often worry that they have *halitosis* or bad breath, and this can seriously affect someone's confidence and quality of life. Often, these folks are obsessed with cleaning their teeth, and frequently they use oral care products that are not helpful, because they are either acidic or mouth-drying, which can make the situation worse. No one with an acidic or dry mouth will ever find relief from halitosis by brushing and flossing, even if they do so ten times per day. This is because the problem is an imbalance in their mouth ecology, and constant cleaning, rinsing, and flossing—especially with aggressive antiseptics or antibacterial products—will only create a more destabilized situation and more embarrassment, expense, and frustration.

Scorched-earth tactics are common in dentistry, which is why patients assume it is correct to scrape the tongue or use prescription products for bad breath. When you appreciate the delicate bacterial balance in our mouths, which includes our tongues, you understand why scraping and killing will not promote the desired outcome. Consider the coral reef analogy, and remember that planktonic or floating microbes will never be controlled by scraping or flossing. The mouth ecology communicates with the nose, ears, and throat, and it may be more useful to consider the health of these areas and add a xylitol nasal spray to your daily xylitol regimen if you suspect allergies or postnasal drip could be involved in your halitosis problems.

Don't sabotage your mouth health by trying to eliminate all your mouth bacteria, because this could allow yeasts or aggressive mouth pathogens an opportunity to develop. The best approach is to minimize periods of acidity in your mouth and develop habits—like ending meals with xylitol—that will frequently alkalize your mouth. Selecting oral care products is always difficult, but this daily mouth care routine must be an integral part of your strategy for a balanced and healthy mouth.

Research in 2007 by V. Haraszthy et al. from the University of Buffalo, and research in 2010 by Takeshita in Japan looked at the relationship between oral malodor and bacteria found on the tongues and in the saliva of people with and without bad breath. These studies showed that the bacteria of people with halitosis was distinct, especially the bacteria on the top surface of their tongues. These bacteria and the bacteria found in saliva were different from bacteria found on the tongues and in saliva of people with inoffensive breath. They also noted that their mouths had limited bacterial diversity. In other words, these sufferers had the opposite of a healthy ecology. In the case of halitosis, there is often an initial bacterial upset following antibiotic exposure or a digestive upset, and then the vulnerable ecosystem can be further exacerbated by any allergies, chronic sinus or nasal problems, acidity from the stomach or throat, or even constant cleanings with incorrect products.

Many people with bad breath do not like the taste of water, and some are almost addicted to soda drinks and juices. Unfortunately, even diet or sugar-free versions of these acidic drinks perpetuate an unhealthy ecology and create conditions that favor periodontal pathogens and other harmful mouth bacteria. Some of these bacteria secrete liquid poisons or toxins, which can become dissolved in any water that you drink, giving it a foul taste. When children or adults say that they do not like the taste of water, consider mouth health may be part of their taste problem. My strategies for mouth health, which we will discuss fully in chapter 9, can usually eliminate harmful mouth bacteria in about twelve weeks and potentially enable you to enjoy drinking water again.

The first step to stop bad breath is to control periods of mouth acidity, and if you are addicted to soda, try to drink it only at meals, and finish the meal with xylitol gum or mints to alkalize your mouth. Don't allow yourself soda outside mealtimes, and if you need to drink between meals, try water sweetened with some xylitol. To make this, add 1 teaspoon of granular xylitol to 3 cups of room-temperature water, and when the granules have dissolved, you can refrigerate this xylitol water, and the xylitol will remain dissolved. Xylitol will not dissolve in cold water. Remember, you will not have the same benefits from drinking xylitol dissolved in water as from a mint or piece of gum. This is because xylitol's hygroscopic effects are nullified by dissolution in the water. Drinking xylitol water can still be useful, especially for people with halitosis, and it can be an alternative to sweet or acidic drinks as your taste buds learn to appreciate the taste of water again.

Combatting Bad Breath
Following are my top six suggestions for combatting bad breath:

1. Control mouth acidity by eating xylitol mints or gum, especially after *every* meal, snack, or drink.

2. Clean your toothbrush every time you use it, and allow it to air-dry—away from any toilet—for twenty-four hours between uses.

3. Stop drinking—even water—for at least a few hours in the afternoon.

4. Follow my Complete Mouth Care System twice or three times (maximum) daily. Do not overclean your tongue or mouth.

5. If you travel, take inexpensive throwaway brushes. Never store a brush in a bag or under a cover.

6. Try to improve your digestive health by including a wide variety of vegetables in your diet, and consider if digestive enzymes and colon probiotics could improve your nutritional status and the quality of your saliva.

7. Foods that boost your immune health include mushrooms, onions, garlic, and pomegranate. Try adding small amounts of these foods to at least one meal each day.

ORAL CARE PRODUCTS

Today, we are faced with an incredible selection of pastes, rinses, and products for tooth care. Many products claim to stop sensitivity, whiten teeth, and prevent bad breath, yet the oral health of America continues to deteriorate. The problem is that few of these products are designed for oral health, but instead they are targeted as a temporary fix for the superficial symptoms. For example, they may give you instant minty breath, less sensitivity, or whiter teeth—but the real solution is to control the underlying problems of an imbalanced or diseased mouth. Of course, toothpaste companies are trying to give you, the consumer, what *you* want. However, it's important to realize that the kind of toothpaste you put on your toothbrush is important as it can help or harm your efforts to achieve oral health.

Toothpaste marketing is alluring, so be sure you are an educated shopper. A toothpaste's ideal ingredients would be nonabrasive silica, enough sodium fluoride to strengthen teeth, and no glycerin. In the late 1950s, the original Crest formulation passed randomized clinical trials and showed it could stop cavities before they start, which means it was shown to prevent cavities. It has been my toothpaste of choice for three decades, despite the fact it contains color and some ingredients I wish were not there. A good toothpaste has value, especially when it is combined with effective brushing techniques. A toothbrush cannot strengthen your teeth or heal a cavity, but the toothpaste that you put on your brush *can* contribute to this process if it contains ingredients that stimulate remineralization and tooth healing. If your mouth is not as you want it to be, consider your toothpaste, and make a simple change.

If your teeth are pristine, healthy, and have never had a single cavity, filling, sealant, or crown at any time in your life, you probably have a wide selection of toothpastes that will work for you. You may enjoy one that contains activated charcoal, one that is chocolate-derived, xylitol gel, or xylitol crystals sprinkled on a damp toothbrush. These are choices that do no harm, and they are also good choices for children who are at no risk for cavities.

On the other hand, if you have gum recession, be sure to avoid any toothpaste that contains glycerin, salt, peroxide, coconut oil, or baking soda, since these can upset biofilm health by dissolving its foundational proteins. If you have a dry mouth or sensitivity, my advice is to avoid all the pastes advertised for sensitive teeth and dry mouth and consider the strategies in this book that address mouth acidity and tooth demineralization problems. Many mouth rinses are acidic, which can make your mouth feel as if they are covered in wool, and they can also cause teeth to become brittle. If you have had fillings in any tooth—even years ago— you will need a toothpaste that can help repair the microscopic enamel cracks that occur on the sides of these teeth. If your mouth needs help, or if it is sensitive or dry, or if you have already had one or more fillings, be sure to consider using xylitol and my Complete Mouth Care System, which helps to strengthen your teeth and will stop enamel from chipping around fillings and from the sides of your teeth.

DAILY MOUTH CARE

Ninety-five percent of people living in the United States have infected mouth biofilm. These people can probably identify the substance known as plaque on their teeth and may have even noticed it as a white foamy material, which is actually biofilm heavily infected with harmful mouth bacteria. Statistics show that a trained hygienist who carefully brushes and flosses teeth can only remove 40 percent of infected plaque from someone's mouth. This is because the remaining 60 percent of problematic bacteria are floating in saliva or attached to other areas of the mouth, nose, or throat, which are inaccessible to a toothbrush. Brushing and flossing cannot turn bad bacteria into healthy ones, which is why we need a new approach.

At night, our mouths become drier than during the day and everyone's saliva becomes more acidic. This makes the night a high-risk time for everyone's teeth, which is why it is vital to adequately prepare your mouth before sleeping. Before bed, I recommended preparing your mouth for this difficult time. My routine can help anyone with weak teeth, dry mouth, darkening teeth, or sensitivity. If you feel you are at risk for cavities or gum problems or if you are someone with a dry mouth, here are four basic suggestions:

1. Use the Complete Mouth Care System described in chapter 9 twice daily and always before sleeping at night.
2. Disinfect your toothbrush, and allow it to air-dry for twenty-four hours between uses.
3. Use xylitol to protect your teeth after every meal, snack, and drink.
4. Give your teeth as much time as possible to interact with saliva, especially during the afternoon. Drink mainly at mealtimes and control sipping (even water), which dilutes saliva's supersaturated status and will reduce its healing power.

CHAPTER 7

Oral Care for Children and Teens

An ounce of prevention is worth a pound of cure.
—Benjamin Franklin

There are some dental truths that may be new to you, and some of these may sound shocking if you have always believed a different story. It's important to know the facts, and so I will try to dispel the most frequent myths and explain the relevance of understanding the truth. The four questions we will explore are:

1. Does sugar attack teeth?
2. How do you "clean" teeth to be cavity-free?
3. Do baby teeth influence adult oral health?
4. Are cavities genetic, and are they preventable?

You could try to answer these questions now and then compare your thoughts after you have learned more about these topics. Hopefully this chapter will give you more confidence and knowledge to effectively care for your children's teeth.

TRUTH 1: SUGAR DOES NOT ATTACK TEETH— BUT IT FEEDS TOOTH-DAMAGING BACTERIA.

You can soak a tooth in sugar, and nothing will happen. Sugar exerts its tooth-damaging effect by providing fuel and conditions that are ideal for harmful bacteria to grow and multiply on teeth. Cavity-forming bacteria produce acids, which soften teeth and create an entry place into the tooth, where they will continue to destroy the tooth's structure and form cavities. Since xylitol behaves in the opposite way from sugar, it can be wiped on teeth or eaten frequently as mints or gum to help rid the mouth of cavity-forming plaque bacteria and to deprive the harmful bacteria of the energy they require to grow, multiply, or stick to teeth.

Because bacteria are fueled by even tiny amounts of sugar, as the consumption frequency of any sugar or carbohydrate increases, so does the risk for tooth damage. Conversely, as the frequency of xylitol exposure increases, the more beneficial are its effects to control harmful plaque bacteria and promote healthy ones. Toddlers often eat small amounts of fruit, bread, cookies, and snacks. All these foods—no matter how healthy and organic they are—digest to become sugary liquids in the mouth, and it is this sugary liquid that fuels harmful bacteria. These damage-promoting conditions continue for up to an hour after eating carbohydrates or sugars, but a clever strategy is to end snacks and meals with a tooth-protective food or xylitol. Tooth-protective foods help control mouth acidity but xylitol additionally works to promote good bacteria and rid the mouth of cavity-forming ones.

TAKEAWAY:

- It is more practical to control the bacterial composition of a child's mouth than try to completely eradicate all forms of sugar and carbohydrates in a child's diet, which is not a realistic option.
- Every exposure, even tiny amounts of sugar or carbohydrates in any form, fuels the growth of cavity-forming bacteria and increases the chance of tooth damage.
- Xylitol alkalizes the mouth and helps control cavity-forming plaque bacteria, which can dramatically lower a child's risk for cavities.
- It is good to limit sugar and carbohydrates in our diet, but frequency of sugar exposure determines the severity of the tooth damage more than the total amount of sugar consumed.
- Frequent tiny amounts of xylitol will more effectively reduce harmful bacteria than a larger amount consumed at one time.

TRUTH 2: YOU CANNOT "CLEAN" TEETH TO BE BACTERIA-FREE, BUT YOU CAN PROMOTE A CAVITY-FREE MOUTH BY NURTURING HEALTHY BACTERIA.

Although we want to control harmful bacteria, we do not want to sterilize our mouth. A mouth devoid of bacteria is not healthy. A healthy mouth is naturally filled with a wide diversity of beneficial bacteria that work to protect it and keep it free from harmful kinds that cause disease and cavities. Destroying healthy bacteria in the mouth will limit this protection and damage the mouth's ecosystem, which is the backbone of true mouth health. Exposure to a variety of bacteria will benefit infants and children and it means we should encourage kissing and contact with adults and other family members. The key is to exchange healthy bacteria with your infants and children and try to limit their exposure to harmful ones. Children whose mouths are populated by a healthy selection of oral bacteria will grow up to enjoy attractive natural teeth that gleam in sunshine and sparkle as they smile.

You should not aim to physically clean all bacteria from teeth, and adding probiotic supplements is not a solution either. The mission should be to use a progressive and effective strategy that nurtures a wide diversity of healthy bacteria in your child's mouth, ideally starting at the moment a first tooth erupts. Try to replace the idea of cleaning teeth with a new idea of nurturing your child's overall mouth health.

—

In the 1970s, pure xylitol chewing gum was given to pregnant women who had bad teeth, and these women had cavities that were never treated, because they lacked access to dentistry. These women were able to improve the bacterial composition of their mouths and minimize their levels of cavity-forming bacteria by 98 percent, simply by eating a few grams of xylitol each day. These mothers kissed their babies after they were born and transferred healthier oral bacteria to their children. At six years old, these children had 85 percent less tooth decay than the children whose mothers did not chew xylitol gum. Traditional dental advice in the United States is for mothers to avoid sharing their mouth bacteria with their children by sterilizing toys and not kissing their babies on the lips. This cannot be recommended for the medical, emotional, or dental health of the child. The baby's mouth *will* become infected with bacteria, arriving from *someone* or *somewhere*. So, if you are pregnant or a young mother, take action and consider improving your own mouth health so that you can share healthier bacteria with your baby. You can also wipe your baby's teeth with a few grains of granular xylitol 3–5 times each day. Xylitol will nurture healthy mouth bacteria and loosen any plaque that may have infected your baby's mouth.

TAKEAWAY:

- You do not need to fight a small child to floss or brush their teeth. Give them xylitol treats, or let them suck on a clean toothbrush dipped in a few xylitol crystals instead.

- Focus on ways to adjust eating and drinking habits to promote healthy bacteria and not harmful ones that feed on sugar and carbohydrates.

- Try to limit snacking and nibbling on sugary or acidic foods, and snack instead on the tooth-protective foods outlined in chapter 4 when possible.

- Don't listen to out-of-date recommendations that tell you to avoid kissing your children. You intuitively know such ideas are wrong. Xylitol is your ally. Learn how to use it in your family. Healthy teeth at age four are a good indicator of a child's future oral health.

TRUTH 3: BABY TEETH ARE VITAL AND INFLUENCE ADULT ORAL HEALTH.

Some people think baby teeth fall out and so these little teeth are of little or no importance, but this could not be further from the truth. Baby teeth play a vital role in the development of a child's future mouth ecology, and this can determine his or her oral health as an adult. The bacteria that cover a first baby tooth as soon as it erupts will provide the foundation for the child's future oral health. Bacterial sharing is continuous between adults and children throughout life, as we interact with, cuddle with, or kiss one another. Bacteria will easily transfer from an adult's mouth to a baby's mouth, and the first bacteria to cover a child's tooth will easily transfer to consecutive teeth as others erupt alongside. An infant's mouth ecology will continue to develop as the child matures, and many kinds of good and bad bacteria will reach a baby's mouth in the first years.

The kind of bacteria that thrive in your baby's mouth will be the ones that benefit by the foods and drinks that he or she is consuming. During the first years of life, it is relatively easy to control the kinds of bacteria that will flourish and become dominant in your baby's mouth. This offers you an amazing opportunity to help a young child develop a wonderful and diverse bacterial ecology that can be the foundation for a lifetime of oral health.

As baby molars erupt, you have one of *the most important opportunities* of all to affect the future mouth health of your child. The bacteria that are the first to cover these new molars will gain a foothold in their grooved biting surfaces. The kind of bacteria that gain entry to these grooves will begin to dominate the mouth's ecosystem. Preparing your child's mouth to be as healthy as possible before these baby molars erupt is a simple way to promote the future mouth health of your child. These baby molars erupt soon after a baby's first birthday, but there are some other opportunities that are almost as powerful for change: during kindergarten (as first permanent molars erupt), in the teen years from

---

TAKEAWAY:

- You cannot stop bacterial transfer, which is a totally desirable and normal part of healthy development. The sooner you guide your child's mouth ecosystem, the easier it will be to establish *healthy bacteria* in the molar grooves, where they will become entrenched and offer protection *from* cavities, potentially for a lifetime.

- There are a few easy steps that can help pregnant mothers, grandparents, and parents to prepare their mouths for sharing *healthy* bacteria with children in the family. It is important to comprehend that, although fillings may be necessary to fix damage,

continued

> fillings do not bacterially improve the health of your mouth.
>
> - Xylitol should offer encouragement to every family with bad teeth, because it offers a way to change the mouth's ecosystem from unhealthy to healthy over a six-month period. Regular use of xylitol has been shown to help prevent the transfer of harmful cavity bacteria to the next generation and to other children in a family, no matter the previous family history of cavities or bad teeth.

eleven to twenty-one years of age (when premolars and molars erupt), and finally in the college years (as wisdom teeth erupt).

TRUTH 4: CAVITIES ARE NOT GENETIC AND ARE COMPLETELY PREVENTABLE.

Bad teeth are not a genetic trait, like a pointy nose or small ears, passed down the family tree. Genetics can affect oral health if a hereditary feature creates an increased risk for cavities. Like any other risk, this can be overcome with strategies designed to protect teeth and avoid dental problems. Remember, oral bacteria are transferable and literally pass from one generation to the next in droplets of saliva, moving from person to person as we kiss and interact with each other and even as we use toothbrushes. Children who develop healthy oral bacteria will have protection from cavities and gum disease and vice versa. The truth is that an inherited family feature may put you at increased *risk* for developing cavity-forming bacteria in your mouth or increase your susceptibility for bad teeth, which can make the dental problems *appear* to be genetic.

Hereditary features create risks for teeth, because they promote either acidic or dry mouth conditions, which are ideal for plaque-forming bacteria. Families may share a similar face, nose, or mouth structure that predisposes them to allergies, sinus problems, or mouth breathing, which all create drier mouth conditions. Certain jaw or lip shapes can make it difficult for people to seal or close their mouths and moisten their front teeth with saliva. Any of these features promote an environment preferred by cavity disease bacteria. This is why inherited features shared by family members can put an entire family at increased risk for cavities and dental disease.

TAKEAWAY:

- You or your children may be at a higher *risk* for cavities, because you are a mouth breather, have allergies, crowded teeth, or incomplete lip closure, but you can gain control over your mouth's ecology and overcome these risks.

- Xylitol stimulates a flow of alkaline saliva into the mouth and can help control a dry mouth when used regularly. Xylitol will also help improve the ecology of your mouth and reduce the number of harmful bacteria to limit your risk for cavities. Xylitol works as the centerpiece of my Complete Mouth Care System, which offers cavity protection from the time adult teeth begin to erupt at around six years of age.

- If allergies, nasal drip, or sinus issues are compounding your dental problems, consider the additional use of a xylitol nasal spray, since it works to clear the nasal passages as effectively as xylitol clears and promotes health in the mouth.

PREVENTIVE CARE DURING PREGNANCY AND AFTER DELIVERY

The womb was believed to be a sterile environment, but now we know this is not accurate. Bacteria have been discovered in the placenta and also in the amniotic fluids around the baby. We also know that a mother's mouth health can directly influence the health of her unborn baby's initial gut bacteria. As a result, pregnant women should work to establish their own mouth health even before their babies are born.

Also, just before birth, hormonal changes alter the mother's body pH and create an alkaline medium, friendly to healthy bacteria, in the mother's vagina. This coats the baby as he or she passes headfirst through the birth canal. Dentists have often observed that children born by cesarean section appear more likely to have cavities. A cesarean-delivered baby may be more easily infected by harmful bacteria after birth and may also be more likely to experience colic, acid reflux, and stomach acidity than vaginally delivered children. Xylitol can easily be used to reverse any negative oral health consequences from cesarean-section birthing.

Breast Milk

Breast milk is a very misunderstood topic, and it frustrates me that breastfeeding has so often been thought a *cause* of early childhood caries. Media headlines have distorted the truth with false emphasis, and often the studies do not reflect the meaning of the headline. This was the case in a newspaper headline that falsely claimed that breastfeeding causes cavities.

In 2005, a study at the University of Rochester was published in the local paper with the headline: "Breast Milk Causes Cavities." I immediately read the study, which was done on rats and did not deliver this result at all. I complained to the newspaper editor and the lead researcher, asking them to correct this error, which they eventually did, but the damage had been done.

Breast milk will only cause cavities if the baby's mouth has been infected and allowed to develop very harmful plaque, an anaerobic kind that can ferment milk. Mothers should avoid passing harmful cavity bacteria to their babies, and they should also wipe erupting baby teeth with xylitol to clean them daily and ensure that they are not coated with unhealthy, stagnant plaque. Provided the baby's mouth is protected in this way, breast milk will *not* cause cavities.

A baby with *healthy* mouth bacteria can safely drink breast milk from a bottle or be breastfed *even* during the night, and you will *not* need to immediately wipe or clean the baby's teeth after this night feeding. A healthy mouth, with balanced and healthy bacteria is *not at risk*. The only risk is when aggressive anaerobic plaque bacteria are present, since they can ferment the milk and create strong lactic acids, which damage the baby's teeth. These bacteria take days and even weeks to grow, and they are easily and quickly removed with some xylitol on a soft cloth or brush. Your baby will not need surgery for a lip tie, and do not allow yourself to be blamed for giving the baby a bottle or breastfeeding as a cause of dental problems. It is not pooling milk that is the concern but, rather, the pooling of cavity bacteria. Remember to wipe the hidden areas of your baby's teeth that are close to the gumline every day with some xylitol; then, you can nurse your child with confidence, even when he or she has multiple teeth during the second year of life.

Remember, acidic or sweetened juices *do* cause problems to teeth directly by their acidity. Baby formula and skim milk are also *not as safe as breast milk*, although cleaning teeth with xylitol reduces cavity risks. Feed any acidic tooth-damaging drinks at mealtimes, and try to wipe the teeth afterward with xylitol, or as your child grows, consider giving him or her a xylitol mint or xylitol gum after meals. For mothers who have problems weaning children from juice in a sippy cup, try to interrupt the duration of sipping with tooth-safe snacks of very tiny cheese cubes to help break the damaging cycle of juice drinks.

SEALANTS

Sealants may give temporary protection to the most vulnerable biting surfaces in molar teeth, but there are alternative strategies that are equally effective and can help you avoid the potential hazards of placing sealants in your child's teeth. Parents looking for protection for their children's teeth have a choice: seal up the grooves of molar teeth and try to block out all bacteria, or adopt a long-term approach that works to nurture healthy bacteria and encourage them to colonize the molar grooves and dominate your child's mouth. It takes about six months of adequate amounts of xylitol to adjust a mouth's ecology—to promote good bacteria and eliminate unhealthy ones. Xylitol offers a natural defense system and one that will continue to offer long-term and more sustainable benefits than sealants, especially when xylitol is consumed regularly before and during times of tooth eruption.

Remember that sealants are a type of plastic, and even those sealants said to be free of BPA are also plastic and will require constant maintenance to prevent the problems that occur if they chip or break and allow liquids to seep under the sealant surface. Most important of all, sealants make it impossible to visually check the mouth and determine any change in health, taking away the ability for advance warning that can alert you to potential decay in these grooves. Losing sight of the molar grooves obliterates these bellwethers of mouth health, and now you only have one option: depend on regular X-rays for the rest of your child's life to determine if cavities have formed.

—

One day, a friend told me that his dentist wanted to put sealants on his son's teeth, and he had insisted that, without sealants, these teeth would become severely decayed by the boy's next six-month checkup. I explained to the family how to improve the mouth's ecology, using xylitol to promote healthy bacteria, and a dilute 0.05 percent sodium fluoride rinse to hasten mineralization and maturation of the new six-year-old molars. We discussed diet and healthy snacking and how a cavity usually takes over a year to form, but often can be reversed in a matter of months. With this approach, the motivation for a sealant was removed. The dentist checked the child's teeth six months later, and found healthy molar grooves. The boy's mouth health had improved, and his risk for decay had disappeared without the need for any dental treatments.

BLEACHING CHILDREN'S TEETH

A relatively new craze is causing damage that may not be fully recognized for decades. Sadly, it almost seems normal today to artificially whiten teeth. However, many studies indicate that this may not be safe, especially for the newly erupted teeth of seven- or eight-year-old children. These newly erupted teeth are delicate and start their life in the mouth lacking minerals, which is why they usually look darker at first. Artificially whitening young teeth may make them look whiter but minerals are lost in the process. Bleaching can also damage the internal proteins, damage the surrounding gums, and weaken a tooth's outer enamel.

New adult teeth erupt into the mouth only partially mineralized, which means their enamel is soft and very porous. Light does not reflect properly on their surface until they have fully mineralized and hardened, which may take from six to twelve months through a natural process called *maturation*, which allows the new teeth to absorb minerals into their outer layer. Until this mineralization process has been completed, these teeth will always appear dull or yellowish in color, especially in stark contrast to the extreme white color of most baby teeth.

These new adult teeth are soft and easily stained and can be at risk for tooth decay. As a pediatric dentist, I believe the last thing these new teeth need is to be whitened with commercial whitening toothpastes that are abrasive or with whitening rinses or treatments that may make the new teeth look white but actually damage these teeth, roughen their surfaces, and pull out minerals that can cause enamel erosion, sensitivity, and a higher risk for cavities. Many studies have warned of the dangers to the protein structure of teeth following whitening, and this is an even bigger concern for thin, young enamel, which is very vulnerable. Nerve and pulp damage can sometimes lead to the death of the tooth—not immediately, but possibly in the future—and there is legitimate concern that changes to the stem cells inside a tooth could trigger blood problems many years ahead.

The most logical approach to help new teeth appear whiter is to be sure they are given every chance to mineralize. This would include careful habits, a good diet that includes healthy fats, adequate protein and possibly bone broth, plus a regimen of daily xylitol. You may want to consider vitamin supplements and digestive probiotics for a limited time as part of your child's daily routine. Keep acidic drinks, particularly carbonated drinks and juices, to mealtimes. A dilute 0.05 percent sodium fluoride rinse will hasten the mineralization process, and the Complete Mouth Care System that I recommend in chapter 9 will quickly help to improve the color of these teeth.

Please ensure that your child rinses and spits effectively. At first, your child may need guidance to ensure he or she uses each rinse in the correct order and does not rinse with water between the steps. You may want to take photos and monitor the progress as these teeth gradually whiten over a period of about two years. The system I suggest will stimulate natural mineralization, as it encourages minerals from saliva to enter the teeth. Xylitol promotes a healthy mouth ecology and also helps control mineral loss from teeth. My mouth rinse system promotes conditions that stimulate mineralization, and the less teeth demineralize and the more teeth mineralize, the whiter they will look.

FLUORIDE: PROS AND CONS

Fluoride is not a vitamin, and parents need to know that I do not recommend fluoride as a supplement or as an additive to drinking water, because dental prevention does not depend on fluoride being absorbed into the body. *Ameloblasts* are cells found in the jaws of infants and babies, and these cells produce the material that forms a tooth's outer enamel shell. Ironically, it is these enamel-forming ameloblasts that are most sensitive to, and most easily damaged by, ingested fluoride. If these cells are harmed by fluoride, the teeth will continue to grow, but gaps occur where enamel does not form properly. These enamel defects are seen as white spots or, in more severe cases, brown spots.

This condition is known as *fluorosis*, and this damage is only possible during the development stage as teeth are forming in a baby's jawbone. Fluorosis is only possible if a child *ingests* too much fluoride between birth and three years of age. This is why children under the age of six should avoid *any consumption* of fluoride in their water or diet. I feel strongly about artificially fluoridated water, and I believe that other less visible health issues may occur alongside the fluorosis of teeth. I also believe that girls are more adversely affected than boys by the consumption of fluoride. On the other hand, I view the appropriate use of topical fluoride (in pea-size amounts of toothpaste or a 0.05 percent dilute fluoride rinse) as helpful for mineralizing newly erupted adult teeth or teeth that, in certain circumstances, have decay and are at risk for needing fillings. Children younger than six should not need to use any fluoride products.

Fluoride—My Personal Story

My five children were born between 1977 and 1990. I had been trained to believe in fluoride, so I gave my first child fluoride drops in the recommended concentration, because I lived in an area without fluoride in the water. At that time, dentists believed that giving fluoride to infants would allow their teeth to grow more perfectly, with smoother surfaces and more resistance to decay. My first daughter's two permanent front teeth erupted, and they had large brown marks in the center enamel of each. Her ameloblast cells had been poisoned by the fluoride drops I added to her water each day when she was a baby. The damage was not visible until these adult teeth erupted at age eight. To correct their appearance, she later required cosmetic dental repair with veneers to mask the damage.

I gave slightly less fluoride to my second daughter, who was born in 1979, because I was a busy mother. This daughter has less damage, but all her teeth are covered in cloud-like spots on the front and side teeth, the result of similar (but slightly less) poisoning of her enamel-producing cells. Both of these daughters have evidence of thyroid damage, but not my other children, who never received fluoride supplements. My family filters fluoride out of our drinking water, and my grandchildren are never given any fluoride to drink. On the other hand, since the age of about six (when they could rinse and spit), my children have used a dilute sodium fluoride rinse twice per day, as part of the Complete Mouth Care System, which has protected their teeth and kept them healthy and cavity-free.

The use of topical fluoride cannot cause fluorosis, since fluorosis only occurs when fluoride is ingested during the period when teeth are developing—before the age of three.

Fluoride Varnish

As a child's first permanent molars erupt during kindergarten or first grade, there will be no sign of a loose or missing tooth as they erupt behind the row of baby teeth at the back of the mouth. These molars are vulnerable to decay in an infected mouth and often have cavities within a year of eruption. Up to 93 percent of these first permanent molars have decay within two years of erupting, and pediatric dentists are accustomed to treating children who need crowns, root canals, or even extraction of these new adult teeth, even before they have had time to fully mineralize and harden. This is why the preschool and kindergarten years are the perfect time to start using xylitol to improve a child's mouth health. To speed mineralization of any new adult teeth, a tiny amount of sodium fluoride toothpaste can be brushed on the outside of these emerging teeth to encourage maturation and to strengthen the enamel to offer maximum protection from decay. If one of these new molars has poorly formed enamel or a soft spot, your dentist may suggest a fluoride varnish as a way to help protect this tooth. A fluoride varnish is a resin that is painted onto teeth, and it will stick to teeth for a month or two. Don't confuse a fluoride varnish with a plastic sealant or with the goopy fluoride gels or foams that are sometimes applied to teeth but which have little or no benefits. A fluoride varnish applied to newly erupted teeth, combined with the daily use of xylitol, is a good suggestion, since it offers some direct help to prevent cavities and may speed up tooth maturation, allowing these new teeth to gain their natural and unique protective covering more quickly. When the fluoride varnish wears off, the tooth remains pristine and unharmed, and there is no blocking of the grooves or damage to the tooth surface.

Basically, this approach is just another way to combine xylitol with sodium fluoride, as I suggest in my home care regimen. Fluoride rinsing definitely helps hasten tooth mineralization and maturation, which will increase the odds that your child's new tooth will remain cavity-free for life. It is difficult to say if varnish offers any more benefit than a 0.05 percent sodium fluoride home rinse. I think the choice depends on each family situation.

If you have difficulty monitoring your child's regular routines, a dentist-applied fluoride varnish may be an advantage and a convenient option to help speed up the absorption of minerals by the young enamel of this newly erupted tooth. To ensure good daily use of my Complete Mouth Care System, you will need to oversee your child's bedtime routine, and if these events are not well orchestrated, it may be prudent to have some extra help from a fluoride varnish rather than end up needing a filling in the future.

Fluoride Rinsing

Only children who can safely spit should use a fluoride rinse. If your young child needs the healing help of fluoride because they have damaged teeth, I recommend either brushing your child's teeth with a good fluoride toothpaste or asking your dentist about coating on a fluoride varnish. Before you allow a child to use a fluoride rinse, have them practice using plain water to determine if they can rinse and spit safely.

I suggest parents slowly add a drop or two of the fluoride rinse to a small cup of water, adding more as the child's ability to rinse and spit improves. Eventually, you will build to a full-strength and undiluted rinse. Most of us need to spit at least twice (one spit followed immediately by another spit) to effectively remove the fluoride rinse from our mouths. Encourage your young child to spit several times, because extra spitting is fun and also ensures they do not hold rinse in their mouths and swallow it. Do not use any other rinse, and try not to let the child eat or drink after the fluoride rinse for about an hour or longer. This is why the perfect moment to use this rinse is just before bedtime.

Fluoride Toothpaste

For children who are at risk for cavities or who have cavities, I recommend a pea-size amount of a plain fluoride toothpaste, a paste that contains some sodium fluoride and silica and does not contain any *glycerin or glycerol*, an ingredient which could hinder the mineralization process. Some toothpaste is too abrasive, and I never recommend any paste with whitening agents, baking soda, or tartar-control chemicals, or any paste designed for sensitivity.

Twelve-year molars and wisdom teeth are as vulnerable as any new teeth when they erupt into a teenager's mouth. These later-erupting molars frequently cause problems, because they are at the back of the mouth and difficult to clean. With my own children, I discovered that xylitol and the Complete Mouth Care System was able to help them successfully erupt these teeth and keep them clean and healthy. Again, parents may need to look for new teeth as they erupt and help their children learn how to brush around them effectively, as techniques for gum massage need to adapt and will not only help promote tooth health but will also maintain gum health.

Professional Recommendations

Many physicians and dentists still prescribe fluoride tablets to children and continue to believe that fluoride's protection occurs from ingesting fluoride. There are also dentists who have been misinformed and remain fearful that breastfeeding causes cavities. Many parents are told that mechanical tooth cleaning is vital, and some parents struggle to comply, believing that brushing and flossing is the way to their children's oral health. Parents can be calmed and become more effective dental health caretakers by understanding the bacterial nature of dental disease and how to employ the incredible benefits of pure xylitol to promote a healthy mouth ecosystem.

The American Academy of Pediatric Dentistry has a mission to seal every fissure in every tooth in the United States, which seems to me to be a catastrophic idea. Be aware that the kinds of mouth bacteria that are naturally resident in the healthy fissures of molar teeth are usually bacteria that aid in the digestion of carbohydrates and gluten. To block these grooves without adequate reason is to expose a child to the plastic BPA, and, more importantly, potentially eradicate the natural habitat suited for these important bacteria. Our concern should be that sealants can leave children at risk for gluten intolerance or for digestive problems at some point in their lives.

BRACES FOR ADULTS AND TEENS

Braces and orthodontic appliances make tooth cleaning complicated, they can prevent your lips from closing over your front teeth, and they can cause mouth breathing, which dries your mouth and leaves it at increased risk for gum disease and cavities. Many orthodontists worry about demineralization of teeth, because they have seen how often this damage occurs.

Braces should never be placed in an unhealthy or infected mouth, but this seems to happen all the time. Sometimes parents imagine that the orthodontist will monitor their child's teeth during treatment, but this may not occur regularly, or at all. Anyone considering braces for their child should ensure that their child's mouth health is virtually perfect *before* the first appointment for braces. Braces can usually wait, and if you don't prepare the child's mouth, braces can quickly turn poor dental health into a dental nightmare. Many teeth are scarred by braces, and this scarring forms white spots, which can easily become cavities. Brackets and other equipment often trap bacteria, and in an infected mouth, hidden in difficult places, these aggressive acid-producing bacteria may demineralize teeth and ruin your child's gum health.

A mother recently told me how her thirteen-year-old has been seeing a dentist regularly since she was small. The girl needed a few fillings each year, despite efforts to limit sugar and brush and floss in the way she had been instructed. The dentist put braces on her teeth to straighten them. When the braces were removed two years later, this young girl needed fifteen fillings in her permanent teeth. The mother feels sad and guilty, and with correct care before and during the time in braces, all this could have been completely prevented.

Of course, everyone should limit sugar and carbohydrates, but it is generally more realistic to insist that sweets and damaging drinks are consumed at mealtimes. Then, your child can learn to end every meal, snack, and drink with xylitol to protect their tooth enamel. Twice per day my Complete Mouth Care System can be used, but children will need adult supervision to ensure they spit out the rinses and use them in the correct order. Sometimes interdental brushes may be useful to clean where food is trapped, and these few strategies during orthodontic treatment can help your child avoid dental drama and instead receive praise for great oral care with no signs of bleeding gums, bad breath, scarred enamel, or cavities.

A NEW APPROACH

Statistics in the United States indicate a pandemic of early childhood caries, teens with fillings in over 75 percent of their teeth, and an estimated 50 percent of thirty-year-olds with gum disease who do not even know about it. The statistics show that, by the end of life, our current generation of seniors have few pristine teeth, and 98 percent have had lost teeth, fillings, crowns, implants, bridges, or dentures. Public health efforts have spent money to try to curb dental disease by teaching the public to brush and floss. Cities all over the United States have built state-of-the-art clinics and school-centered mobile units, and many have developed an army of professionals to treat adults and children, yet the problems escalate.

Today, dental disease is the most prevalent of all childhood diseases, and the 2006 MetLife Oral Health Insights Study for Americans shows that our young people are not doing well either. Twenty-four percent of responders ages 18–34 said their gums bled when they brushed; a third said their teeth were loose or discolored; one out of five young adults described their oral health as fair to poor; 15 percent said they had consistently bad breath; and 27 percent of young people between 18 and 34 said they had sensitive teeth that hurt when they drank hot or cold beverages. If we want to step outside these awful statistics, we must develop a new approach.

The strategies I use for adults can be modified for each stage of a child's development, for patients with or without cavities or gum disease. My focus is always to:

- Develop and nurture healthy mouth bacteria with good eating habits and frequent use of xylitol

- Help teeth become strong and shiny by giving them time to interact with saliva and by choosing oral care products that enhance oral health

- Protect teeth as much as possible from acidic damage

Cavities in children's teeth cannot be regarded simply as a statistic. The painful truth is that one or two cavities can easily crescendo into a lifetime of escalating dental problems. Once a filling has been placed in a tooth, the filling will likely need repair or replacement every 5–10 years. Cavities and gum disease are not inevitable. Xylitol can change the ecosystem of a mouth, weeding out unhealthy bacteria while promoting probiotic and protective ones.

Finland changed its public health policy in 1972 to focus its dental health policies on preventive care and away from drilling and filling. Ninety percent of Finnish kindergartens and preschools now offer xylitol gum to children during the school day in a program to adjust the oral microbiome in advance of the eruption of permanent adult molars. The effectiveness of this program has been monitored, and in 2013, the Finnish National Institute of Health and Welfare recommended that all one- to six-year-olds should be given xylitol confectionery after meals and that publicly funded xylitol products should be provided to children to improve their dental health and decrease the cost of public dental care. My belief is that teaching families about the benefits of xylitol for young children could be an effective and very low-tech method that could help us control dental disease in a fun and delicious way in every community.

As we have discussed, a pregnant mother with bad teeth can use xylitol and change the kind of bacteria that she passes to her baby. She can reduce the chance of decay in her child's teeth simply by reducing the number of harmful bacteria in her own mouth by using xylitol. With a transformed mouth, she will transfer healthy, not bad, bacteria to her baby.

Parents-to-be, even those with cavities, should consider using small but frequent exposures to xylitol during pregnancy and throughout the first years of their baby's life (as baby teeth erupt) to interrupt the transmission of cavity bacteria and improve the long-term dental health outcome for their child. This process can be called *share-care*, which indicates an understanding that health benefits are passed along by *sharing* healthy bacteria between family members. Understanding how share-care works should encourage families to enjoy their loving interactions and kissing one another, especially with a new baby.

Children's mouth health is important. By developing healthier mouths, I am hopeful that the next generation may avoid many of the fearful health conditions exacerbated by poor teeth and gums. With continued efforts to inform and educate, I hope people will navigate the confusion of our current oral health approach. It is my hope that you will be able to take this new information to your extended families and friends and, with these effective home strategies, change the outcome and give your kids and grandkids the gift of healthy teeth—for life!

CHAPTER 8

Changing Your Relationship
with Your Dentist

*The doctor of the future will give no medication, but
will interest his patients in the care of the human
frame, diet, and in the cause and prevention of disease.*

—Thomas Edison

Sometimes the truth is painful. Certain observations throughout history have illustrated unexpected flaws in some generally accepted facts of that era. The problem is that often the messengers of these findings caused commotion and were viewed as defiant or disrespectful simply because the new concept conflicted with the accepted mantra of that time. For example, Copernicus was a mathematician and astronomer in the 1500s who was convinced that the sun, not Earth, was at the center of the universe. His ideas were contrary to the accepted opinions of that time, and so he was hesitant to publish his findings for fear of rejection and retaliation.

My hero is Dr. Ignaz Semmelweis, a physician in the mid-nineteenth century who championed hand washing for doctors, certain it was a simple way to save women from death and horrible infection during childbirth. Dr. Semmelweis was ridiculed, ousted by his peers, and eventually confined to a mental asylum, where he died in a straightjacket at the age of forty-seven. Dr. Semmelweis's hand washing strategies offended doctors who held different opinions about disease. He was also unable to visibly illustrate the problem he described, because it was invisible. So he stood alone. The saddest part of the story is that, just fifteen years after his death, microscopes became available and were able to show that the "invisible problem" on the doctors' hands were germs, transferred from autopsy cadavers to birthing women.

POSTPONING DENTAL TREATMENT

Before you run to share the strategies in this book with your dentist, you must realize that the idea you can maintain your own oral health is radical thinking. I know dentists who do not believe cavities or gum disease can reverse or heal naturally, and most hang their practice philosophies on the belief you need to floss and have cleanings every six months. This is why I encourage people to share their stories with one another so that others can gain confidence and escape the expenses and discomfort of avoidable treatments. Before you agree to dental treatments, I suggest you ask if it is possible for you to postpone treatment for a little while—possibly until your next appointment. The idea is to use this delay to implement the healing strategies outlined in this book and specifically in the next chapter.

A cavity normally takes at least a year to form, but it can often be reversed in a matter of months. When it comes to self-care, most professionals think it does not matter which toothpaste or rinse you use. Some have heard Listerine or fluoride are problems, and yet other professionals prescribe stronger versions of these. With such a variety of opinions, whom do you believe?

I often share the story of Helen Rumbelow, the British reporter who wanted flossing advice but tried my system, without flossing, until her next appointment. She kept her changes private as she sat in the dental chair, amused to hear this third-party endorsement of her improved oral health, despite the warnings her dentist's office had given.

Like Helen, why not try to amaze *your* dentist with improved mouth health by using the strategies of my Complete Mouth Care System? Be aware, your dentist may not understand this system of care and may not have any faith in these products, my methodology, or my recommendations. Note that the American Dental Association (ADA) holds the intellectual property on a number of oral care products and has a vested interest in training people to use and believe in *them*. The other concern is that dentists are frequently gifted samples of products to share with patients at the end of their visits. A free gift is not necessarily a good product, and many appear to have the potential to upset your mouth health. One of my clients was persuaded by a free sample to relinquish her loyalty to the original Crest toothpaste that I recommend. This paste had protected her teeth successfully for twenty years, but she switched to one her dentist gave her in a sample gift bag and was horrified when she began developing staining, cavities, bad breath, sensitive teeth, and finally a dry mouth.

Despite the problems of convincing a disbelieving dentist, I will never recommend that you avoid going to see your dentist. You need a dentist to be the evaluator of your progress, to judge how your daily care system is working, and to step in when actual dental work is necessary.

Two pivotal risk factors, acidity and dry mouth, can ruin any healthy mouth. If you have these conditions, try to figure out how they can be controlled to turn your mouth health around. If you have a cavity in a groove on the biting surface of a molar, for example, consider making changes to protect your teeth from acid damage and mouth dryness. Then, use my suggested oral care protocol in the next chapter to prevent this cavity from progressing. With good strategies, you can often mineralize and rebuild the tooth, so the entire cavity will reverse and disappear.

MONITORING YOUR ORAL CARE PRODUCTS

Be aware of the importance of the oral care products you select. If you have dental problems, consider that the products you are using may not be helping you, and perhaps you should discard them. On the other hand, once you have found a way to enjoy sustainable mouth health and avoid dental problems and no longer need cleanings or treatments, stay loyal to your program. I know people who have faithfully used products that made their teeth sensitive, or they developed calculus and plaque, or they continued to endure unhealthy gums and weak enamel, yet they continued to use the same oral care products, because they had once been recommended to them.

These people were incredulous to discover that a small switch in toothpaste or the addition of rinses could quickly change their dental health. If your teeth are not getting stronger, change your toothpaste, and find a more effective system. Everyone should expect their mouth to feel clean and comfortable, and their teeth should feel shiny, glossy, smooth, and slippery. If your teeth feel dry and sandy or rough and dirty, change what you are using, no matter how recommended, natural, or endorsed this product may be. Two months on a good protocol should improve your oral health, so you will feel confident and make a good impression at your next professional visit.

It's important to be enthusiastic about mouth health, and I believe when someone makes changes, they should be encouraged by seeing and feeling positive results. No one wants to limit favorite foods or conscientiously clean their teeth unless the outcome is successful. I feel sorry for people who are told to drink through straws or use peroxide trays on their teeth every night in efforts to control staining or fight gum disease. Dental issues happen whenever you upset the delicate bacterial balance in your mouth. You will know your ecosystem is out of balance if your teeth are sensitive or if they seem vulnerable to cavities, staining, erosion, or fractures. Regular use of the products I recommend in chapter 9, however, should stop these problems, even for someone who has sensitive teeth or a dry, acidic mouth.

A FEW PRECAUTIONS

Earlier in this book, we discussed transfer of bacteria within families. This is an often overlooked concern outside the family circle for anyone who is dating. Teens, young adults, and even seniors should be warned that oral pathogens transfer—no matter your age group—and statistics show that over 50 percent of the population have periodontal disease bacteria, which transfer from one person to another. Other often unrecognized sources of bacterial transfer are shared office phones and the use of contaminated musical instruments. Woodwind and brass instruments can harbor bacteria for weeks after use, leaving them potential reservoirs to transmit disease to others. Research shows woodwind instruments become more contaminated than brass, and clarinets, for some reason, may be the most susceptible.

Today, more dentists are talking to their patients about bacterial transfer, but perhaps we also need to be concerned about bacteria that hang in the air above dental chairs. In the 1980s, I was involved in research on bacterial transfer in dental offices. A few years later, dental offices were instructed to undergo complete overhauls of their sterilization techniques. For the first time, dentists began to wear gloves and masks and use disposable instruments for surgery and injections. These new mandatory guidelines were only instigated after patients were infected during dental treatment.

We cannot see infection in the air or on surfaces, so I believe we need to continue to be vigilant about transfer of disease on dental equipment, in water lines, and through splatter in the air of dental offices. Few people talk about the risk of patient-to-patient transfer, or the potential for inoculating decay from one tooth to another with a spiky dental probe, or the possible movement of pathogens from one infected pocket to another as periodontal assessments are performed. We know dental masks and eyewear are unable to completely protect dentists from splatter sprayed from a patient's mouth during treatment, but what about the risk for a patient?

A Michigan study tested eye shield protection in 1984, using a phantom patient and red dye, and it clearly illustrated how splatter from a patient's mouth sprayed as the drill touched teeth at speeds from 180,000 rpm to 500,000 rpm. Debris was found to travel up to 50 mph, with pieces of filling, tooth, calculus, and, potentially, bacteria hurled into the air with saliva and blood. This should give you pause as you lie horizontal with your mouth open and your nose, eyes, and skin exposed. If you are a parent, have you considered the consequences for a child with a healthy mouth who is next in line after someone with poor oral health?

It may be time for better air quality control in dental offices and systems for healthy mouths to be examined in a separate room from the operatory where cavities and periodontal disease are treated. In the interim, here are three simple things anyone can do to limit their risk of exposure. And even if these steps are not essential, it may be smart to be cautious:

1. Schedule a dental appointment as early in the day and week as possible, ideally after a long weekend when the office air will have settled. Avoid Friday afternoon when office air may be fogged with bacteria.

2. Boost your immune system with a healthy diet and probiotics for several weeks before an appointment.

3. If you are an adult, you may want to prepare your mouth with my Complete Mouth Care System immediately before an appointment and chew a Zellie's mint or gum as you exit the dental office.

CAMBRA

If you want to talk with your dentist about reversing cavities, you need to know about something called CAMBRA. These initials stand for caries management by risk assessment. In 2010, when my first book, *Kiss Your Dentist Goodbye*, was published, CAMBRA was a new idea, and my book was written to explain this concept and why some people are at greater risk for dental problems. In addition, I explain how to overcome these risk factors and control cavities and gum disease to make dental problems stop.

The CAMBRA concept has now emerged more fully and has been incorporated into many dental office protocols. My introduction to CAMBRA science was decades ago through the teaching of Dr. John Featherstone, who is now the dean and professor at the School of Dentistry at the University of California, San Francisco. Dr. Kim Kutch is another dentist who has also worked tirelessly for many years to teach CAMBRA and explain how patients can avoid fillings and reverse cavities.

A CAMBRA dentist may ask a lot of questions about your diet, acid reflux, and habits that could be affecting your oral health. They will search for the source of acidity in your mouth and may measure acid-producing bacteria. All CAMBRA programs that I know center on the use of xylitol, and many have similarities with my Complete Mouth Care System. I am glad the idea of CAMBRA has raised awareness about natural tooth repair and mineralization, but not all CAMBRA home care suggestions are the same. My belief is that many CAMBRA protocols were developed before dentists understood the role of healthy bacteria and the importance of a healthy microbiome, which is easily damaged by strong fluoride, strong antiseptics, or the use of antibiotics.

Much as I support the concept, the following is a list of my personal concerns about CAMBRA:

- CAMBRA testing currently does not measure either healthy bacteria or gum-disease pathogens. CAMBRA testing measures cavity-forming bacteria found in plaque. I prefer strategies that consider the mouth's complete ecosystem and strategies that develop long-term and sustainable tooth *and* gum health.

- CAMBRA programs sometimes suggest a prerinse of bleach, which can eradicate harmful bacteria, but it will also eradicate healthy bacteria. I prefer a prerinse with chlorine dioxide, because it is does not kill healthy bacteria. The released oxygen from chlorine dioxide disturbs anaerobic pathogens but does no harm to the healthy oral ecology.

- Most CAMBRA systems provide stronger fluoride in their pastes and rinses, which I believe can damage healthy mouth bacteria. Stannous fluoride is often the fluoride preferred by CAMBRA dentists, whereas I recommend only sodium fluoride products. Stannous fluoride can cause staining and upset the mouth's ecology and the delicate mouth tissues.

Hopefully, you will find a dentist who believes in reversing cavities and gum disease and who will be excited to help you end dental problems and improve your oral health without unnecessary treatments. You want to find a dentist who does not see themselves as a fixer of damage but someone who is happy and passionate to be your dental health coach and advisor.

Insurance companies may eventually reward this kind of dentist who is motivated by early detection and wants to help you avoid dental problems. Medical insurance companies know about the close links between mouth health and general health and how chronic systemic health problems may be reduced with improved oral health. United Concordia, a dental insurance company, has recently developed teams of Oral Wellness Consultants whose job is to explain the oral-systemic connection to patients and guide them to dental professionals who understand this link. Unless recommended ideas for oral care are able to truly *improve* mouth health, we will never fully recognize the whole-body benefit that a healthy mouth can bring.

It will be more exciting when insurance companies create enough motivation for dentists to use measuring equipment like the Inspektor Research Systems light technology. These devices measure changes in enamel strength, which can be pivotal in detecting potential weakness early to give you enough time to take action and avoid a filling. By measuring tooth hardness with the precision of these systems, your dentist can check for changes in your teeth's mineralization and determine if your teeth are getting stronger and healthier.

A company called Oral DNA has a test called MyPerioPath®, which measures the levels of periodontal bacteria in your saliva. This can alert you if harmful periodontal pathogens are at an unhealthy level, indicating the probability that they are breeding in gum pockets around your teeth. With Oral DNA testing, you'll swish saline in your mouth and then spit the liquid into a test tube. The sample is sent for analysis, and the periodontal bacteria are identified, measured, and displayed as a graph showing levels of specific pathogens that are implicated in gum disease.

Oral DNA testing can identify eleven kinds of bacteria that are causes for concern and give the level of each compared with a black line, considered the generally accepted safe level, for every kind. Any measurement above this line indicates a problem, since these bacteria have been implicated in various health conditions, and some have been associated with chronic inflammation and its health consequences.

Some bacterial testing involves the insertion of a toothpick-shaped piece of absorbent paper into gum pockets around teeth. The paper soaks up fluids and bacteria from the area, and then it is viewed under a microscope to look for harmful bacteria. The problem with this kind of testing is that some harmful bacteria are normal residents of our mouth, and providing their numbers are low, they pose no problem. Concern should arise when harmful bacteria multiply rapidly, and this can be seen in saliva samples. Because of its limited view, samples gathered from a single pocket could cause unnecessary concern.

There is a still a lot to learn about mouth bacteria, but we already have sufficient information to know that we cannot continue to follow old dental mantras. I suggest everyone takes a salivary mouth test for periodontal pathogens along with an oral cancer screening, at least every couple of years. If you have active gum disease, I believe you should consider testing immediately and then monitor your oral health until it is satisfactory and remains stable. For the latest information about salivary testing, please visit my website at www.DrEllie.com.

BECOMING DENTALLY EMPOWERED

To become dentally empowered, I suggest you begin preparing your mouth *before* your next appointment. If you improve your oral ecosystem before a cleaning, you will be able to imagine as you leave the dental chair and pay your bill that healthy bacteria will be ready to populate your teeth and become the main protectors of your mouth. Changing the mouth's ecosystem is a process that takes time (2–6 months) and requires the progressive reduction of harmful microbes alongside the protection and promotion of beneficial ones.

With healthy bacteria in your mouth, you should be able to extend the time intervals between cleanings, which can translate into stronger teeth and improved oral health. Remember, you cannot simply stop having cleanings and hope that your mouth is healthy. Ultimate oral health demands healthy bacteria and daily care that protect your teeth from the harmful consequences of infected plaque, calculus, and gum infections. Your journey to this place is progressive, and although you can take the first steps today, it may be a year or more before your dentist agrees that you no longer need frequent cleanings to maintain mouth health.

There are currently a lot of studies looking at saliva. Healthy, alkaline saliva promotes bacteria that do not produce acids, and it can control undesirable bacteria in various ways and make certain ones inactive. For example, salivary glands accumulate nitrate from the blood and secrete it into the saliva that washes the mouth. Certain mouth bacteria are able to process salivary nitrate (NO_3^-) and turn it into nitrite (NO_2^-). When nitrite comes into contact with acid-producing bacteria, the nitrite becomes a substance that is toxic to them, and this helps eliminate some of the harmful oral bacteria, especially those that cause cavities.

Nitrates generally reach saliva through the absorption of nitrates from our diet, and they are found in a wide assortment of green leafy vegetables and in beets. The more nitrates in saliva, the more saliva will be able to promote and aid the bacteria that use nitrate (denitrifying bacteria). When denitrifying bacteria are plentiful, they will help to control cavity-causing bacteria and help promote mouth health. Humans lack the nitrate reductase enzyme necessary to turn nitrates into nitrites, so we depend on oral bacteria for this benefit. Furthermore, any nitrite we swallow in our saliva reacts with gastric acids in our stomach to create nitric oxide, which can inactivate potential pathogens in the stomach and will also exert positive vasodilatory effects on our circulation and breathing. It appears that today only 10 percent of the US population has healthy, mineral-dense saliva and the nitrate-reducing bacteria that can naturally protect us in these ways.

Some of these healthy denitrifying bacteria are harmed by oral care products like bleach or the strong antiseptic rinse chlorhexidine, which is a often recommended for gum disease. A Swedish study by Joel Petersson et al. examined rats that had been fed a super nitrate-rich diet. Some of these rats had their mouths sprayed with an antibacterial spray, which damaged their oral bacteria, including the denitrifying bacteria. Then, the rats were given a compound known to cause mouth ulcers. Only the rats whose mouths had been sprayed with the special antibacterial compound developed mouth ulcers. Petersson suggests that the spray killed the denitrifying mouth bacteria, and without these bacteria, the rats lacked the protection that the nitrate-nitrite and nitricoxide effect offers to the skin of the mouth. Without the protection normally offered by healthy bacteria, the antibacterial compound was able to cause ulcerations. This shows the value of a healthy mouth ecology and illustrates why people who experience mouth ulcers should look at ways they can nurture more denitrifying bacteria in their mouths. Generally my advice is to begin with regular use of xylitol after meals and drinks, give thoughtful choice to your selection of oral care products, stop tongue scraping or too frequent mouth cleaning, and enjoy a diet that supports salivary health. This would ideally be a diet that includes plenty of green leafy vegetables, beets, mushrooms, garlic, yogurt, butter, and pomegranate juice.

Remember that you dilute your saliva by sipping anything, and this will dilute the protective benefits of saliva. If this is difficult to imagine, consider what would happen if saliva were the same consistency as water. The crystals of tooth enamel would dissolve into the water in the same way that bath salt crystals dissolve in bath water. The benefits of saliva are enhanced when we make teeth more accepting of saliva's minerals. This is achieved with a solution of 0.05 percent sodium fluoride as a rinse used twice per day. The benefit is created as minerals from saliva become attracted to the tooth surface, where they enter and strengthen the enamel.

TALKING WITH YOUR DENTIST

If you visit your dentist every year, you can use this opportunity to talk and ask questions about changes in your mouth, good or bad. If you begin with poor oral health, you should see improvements quickly, and bleeding gums should heal and disappear if you have been massaging your gums and working to improve your digestive and immune health. My strategies are useful for people fighting cavities and gum disease, but they are also useful for people who have fillings, crowns, bridges, implants, or otherwise damaged teeth, especially as they age or begin to take medications that dry the mouth.

People with good teeth will find that my strategies enhance and safeguard their teeth. Shiny teeth become shinier, healthy gums look better, and teeth feel cleaner. Some people are afraid to tell their dentist about their new approach to oral health. Most biologic dentists are adamant that fluoride should never be used, yet they often witness teeth that fracture or have problems that lead to root canals, crowns, bite guards (which are plastic), fillings (which often contain BPA), or the need for artificial whitening. If you are on a downward spiral of treatments, at least consider changing your home care, and remember that the most biologic and natural dentistry is no dentistry *at all*.

The need for ongoing dental treatments should be a reality check for anyone who is working hard to care for their teeth. You deserve to enjoy sustainable oral health without ongoing treatments. Remember that our understanding of oral health has changed radically in the past ten years, and these new concepts about oral health have exciting implications and should offer great hope to everyone. Why be intimidated? Why not give my strategies a try for a few weeks, even if they fly in the face of something like flossing, which may have been recommended to you but has never worked? I hope you surprise yourself and discover there really is a way to enjoy ultimate oral health and that many of these positive changes will happen easily and relatively quickly.

X-RAYS

When I was a child, there were X-ray machines in shoe stores. As we were fitted for a pair of shoes, it was customary to stand in this machine, so the store clerk could take an X-ray of your shoes to check if your toes had adequate room for growth. There was no protection from the X-rays, and because my father had bad feet, he lovingly insisted that my brother and I had lots of pictures taken to avoid ill-fitting shoes. I cringe when I think how many X-rays I experienced as a preteen child. No one knew of any dangers, but when they did, these machines rapidly vanished forever. There are now studies that say X-rays can be harmful and may damage living tissue and promote cancer, yet they continue to be taken regularly in dental offices, sometimes as often as every six months.

In September 2012, the journal *Cancer* published a study showing an association between dental X-rays and meningioma, a common brain tumor. The results were challenged by the ADA, but that same year, the organization created guidelines to limit a patient's exposure to radiation and avoid unnecessary risk from its long-term effects. I have already mentioned how great it would be for more dentists to use equipment capable of measuring small changes in enamel strength. This equipment was introduced years ago and has been used in other countries for over a decade. The benefit is that the measurements tell you about changes in your tooth strength, which allows you to know if your teeth are getting stronger or weaker. This test involves no radiation, because the measurements are by light reflection. The equipment would be able to give us preventive warnings about areas where enamel is softening, without the need for routine bitewing X-rays, the kind that are part of almost every dental checkup appointment today. Unfortunately, the dental industries associated with all the expensive X-ray equipment will continue to lobby and likely block this new technology to keep it away for as long as possible.

Dental X-rays can be divided into two groups: those taken for preventive screening purposes and those used to investigate a specific problem or injury. X-rays taken for screening are used to ensure everything is healthy, and they allow your dentist to evaluate unerupted teeth and the health of bone and roots below the gumline. If you have an unhealthy mouth, plaque and calculus, cavities and fillings, root canals, crowns, implants, bleeding gums, or periodontal pocketing, you will need diagnostic X-rays often, even as much as every six months. If you have a healthy mouth with pristine teeth, a dentist can be quite confident of your mouth health with far fewer X-rays.

With healthy gums and pristine teeth, the need for X-rays to check deeper should be adequate at three- to five-year intervals. Over fifty years, this extension of the time interval from six months to five years could save you over one hundred potentially unnecessary exposures. When all the crevices of molar teeth have been filled by sealants or covered with fillings or dental crowns, this prevents the dentist from being able to visually judge the health of your mouth, as the molar grooves have been eliminated. As a general rule of thumb, pristine teeth will need the fewest X-rays, and this is one reason I strongly oppose the use of sealants, as they increase the need for frequent X-ray assessment for the rest of your life.

LESS IS MORE

Most people have been conditioned to believe that the more cleanings they have, the better their teeth will be. Companies with a vested interest have encouraged this promotion, aided by the insurance industry and marketers who have created dental software and services to promote dental recalls. The idea of regular cleanings is the darling of business consultants who have encouraged dentists to adopt a business idea called *the hygiene model* of dental practice. These dental offices have one or more dental hygienists, who generate a substantial core income from recall cleanings, usually performed before the dentist has examined the patient or anyone has determined if a cleaning is even necessary. A cleaning can remove discolored and infected biofilm (the material that is called plaque) from teeth in an infected mouth, but a dental cleaning has no power or ability to naturally improve or whiten the actual color of healthy teeth. To review this important point: the color or whiteness of teeth is an illusion that is created as light reflects off enamel prisms on the smooth outer surface of healthy enamel, which is covered by a protective protein film.

Dental professionals are trained to have faith in regular cleanings and there are only a few of us voicing concerns about them, questioning if they can be detrimental to people with a healthy mouth. The concern is that a cleaning removes the hardest part of a tooth, a microscopically thin and vitally important layer on the outside of tooth enamel. As most dental practices in the United States were evolving into hygiene-model practices, the existence of this important enamel layer was not recognized. Recently, we have discovered that the outside protective layer is at least ten times thinner than previously thought and may be important to the health of your mouth because of the ionic charge that is carried on its surface.

This new understanding of the situation suggests that frequent cleanings could create sensitivity, disrupt healthy biofilm, and may even leave teeth more vulnerable to cavities and staining. Patients with a dry mouth lack saliva and may have great trouble replacing healthy biofilm after it has been stripped during a routine cleaning, since saliva proteins are the foundation for rebuilding biofilm. This means people with a dry mouth and less saliva could be particularly damaged by frequent cleanings and find that their teeth become ever more sensitive and progressively more at risk for cavities, stains, and fracture with each cleaning.

If you have a dry or acidic mouth, you should make every effort to adjust your mouth health *before* a cleaning, and remember to ask your dentist if you really *need* one. If you do need a cleaning, consider making every effort to establish healthy biofilm before your next cleaning. Your goal is to ideally create long intervals between cleanings and monitor if this helps you to decrease dental problems like sensitivity and tooth fractures.

Another group of patients who should be wary of cleanings are those who have titanium dental implants. With titanium in your jaw, you should be extremely judicious about the frequency of professional cleanings you receive. This is because there is a substantial risk that particles of metal can be scraped off your implant and get into your gum tissue, which could create a new health hazard. So, once you get to a place where you no longer need a regular cleaning, you should be able to keep your teeth and gums healthy by following my at-home protocol and having periodic check-ins with your dentist to assess the level of your oral health.

We also need to be concerned that frequent cleanings could open the door for a healthy mouth to become infected. Many years ago, some US Navy recruits were selected for a study because they had no plaque, healthy mouths, and were cavity-free. Half the group was given a professional dental cleaning, then *all* the recruits were told to rinse with a solution of cavity-forming *S. mutans* bacteria, the bacteria that infect biofilm and form plaque. Then the groups were tested for *S. mutans* salivary levels after the rinse. The outcome was that the group that had received a cleaning tested positive with high levels of *S. mutans*, whereas the group that did *not* have a cleaning did *not* appear to have become infected by the rinse. It appears that removing the protective layer of beneficial biofilm during the cleaning had allowed this group to become vulnerable and be contaminated by the plaque bacteria. This study was conducted over forty years ago and appears to have never been investigated further but was ignored, as if it never took place.

The majority of people in the United States, if tested, would probably find they do need a cleaning, because they have harmful plaque in their mouths, even many who are fastidious and believe that they take good care of their teeth. Cleanings are useful for people who don't have good oral hygiene, who do not care, or who don't want the responsibility of their own oral health. Please understand that, while I suggest you restrict unnecessary cleanings, I do believe everyone needs a dentist to monitor their oral health. This means we may not all need the same treatment. For example, patients who want to improve their own oral health will need different care from those who are happy to leave their oral health in the hands of their dentists and let their insurance pay for as much treatment as possible.

The first group needs effective advice, careful monitoring, and encouragement to reach their ultimate oral health status. Patients who do not want this responsibility will be served well by traditional dental care, which can treat almost every dental symptom as it occurs. For this second group, the dentist will look for problems at each routine examination and fix issues as they happen. In this way, patients can keep their teeth pain-free and looking good for as long as possible, and all they need to do is show up for their dental appointments and pay the bills.

This means that the most important question is whether or not you want to be responsible for your own mouth health. The time has come, in medicine and in dentistry, to recognize we have two kinds of patients: those who want the doctor or dentist to take care of them and those who want to be empowered, take responsibility for and learn about their health, and self-direct their journey for the best possible outcome. This latter group needs up-to-date, complete, and effective advice, regular monitoring, and encouragement to reach and enjoy optimal bodily and mouth health.

For the past seventy years, traditional dentistry has become a care system that caters to the patient who accepts the need for ongoing treatment, cleanings, repairs, and finally the replacement of their teeth after extractions. This system has grown to offer cosmetic reconstruction for damaged teeth and smiles, and finally it is starting to alert patients to the implications of periodontal disease. Unfortunately, if you decide that you want something more, if you want to be empowered and achieve the highest level of oral health possible and avoid disease and its consequences, your biggest problem will be finding a dentist who believes this is possible, who will encourage you, and who will agree that many treatments and cleanings are unnecessary. Initially, you may have to take it on yourself to prove the point with your own achievements. With correct care and nutrition, you should expect to quickly develop and enjoy a mouth free from plaque, calculus, and cavities and avoid any bleeding gums or periodontal disease.

SUPPORT FROM A WELLNESS DOCTOR AND A DENTIST

Many of the people who buy fancy toothpastes are shocked by my simple and unimpressive suggestions for daily tooth care. On the other hand, there are some who cannot believe I suggest products that contain fluoride as an ingredient. This is why it took a while for me to find my first holistic convert: Dr. Marlene Merritt, a dedicated wellness doctor, herbalist, and acupuncturist in Austin, Texas.

Dr. Merritt was gracious when we met, and she listened to my explanations about the impact of oral health on general health. We discussed all the strategies of my system at length, and eventually she was confident enough to try my system herself and suggest it to her office assistant, someone who had prepaid thousands of dollars for impending gum surgery to perform grafting, deep scaling, and periodontal therapy. For several weeks prior to this appointment, Dr. Merritt's assistant diligently used my strategies and the Complete Mouth Care System. When the appointment time arrived, the office assistant sat in the dental chair and was stunned as her dentist described his amazement at her incredible mouth health improvements. He pronounced the treatment was no longer necessary and gave a complete refund.

This was the start of a long relationship with Dr. Merritt and many of her professional contacts in Austin, Texas. She has also introduced numerous practitioners to my method of oral care during her travels across America as she lectures about the many ways we can reduce our risk for chronic inflammation, diabetes, and Alzheimer's.

DAILY HOME CARE

Daily home care is imperative for maintaining oral health. And if you are using the correct system, it should keep your teeth strong, plaque-free, and comfortable between dental visits. If this is not happening, then something is wrong with your daily care. People who experience soft or weak teeth, plaque buildup, or sensitivity should reconsider the products they use daily. My Complete Mouth Care System is a program that will help develop and maintain oral health and assist you in avoiding unnecessary dental treatments to enjoy ultimate oral health.

Anyone who brushes their teeth is spending money on products for daily use anyway, and often people assume expensive products are better than simple ones. On the other hand, homemade toothpaste can seem like a bargain, but it is not if it permits deterioration of tooth enamel, the eventual loss of fillings, gum recession, sensitivity, broken or dead teeth, and other problems that may lead to expensive root canals and crowns. Just because something is "natural" does not mean it is good for your teeth, and in the next chapter, I will share the dangers of many natural things like oil pulling, salt, baking soda, and hydrogen peroxide.

I often ask people how they rate the status of their mouth health. The responses I get indicate that most people have no idea what constitutes mouth health. Some people tell me they have great teeth, because they have white teeth or straight teeth, but I know they have plaque, acidic damage, gum recession, and are probably told to floss at every dental visit. Most people do not understand the signs of disease, and dental disease is painless and invisible, so how do you know if your mouth is healthy?

We can wish for better testing equipment, but for now, ask your dental team to explain what progress they see and if you are doing a good job caring for your teeth. Reducing your need for cleanings is an excellent sign that you are heading in a good direction. In the next chapter, you will learn about my Complete Mouth Care System, which has all the tools you need to begin a journey to improved oral health.

CHAPTER 9

The Complete Mouth Care System

Your present circumstances don't determine where you
can go; they merely determine where you start.

—Nido Qubein

In this chapter, we will explore the specific mouth care strategies that constitute my Complete Mouth Care System. This program has helped thousands of patients improve their mouth health, no matter the state of their mouth or their previous dental history. Most people have remained loyal to the program for years and have attained the goal of sustainable oral health that requires virtually no professional maintenance. Among the achievements are cavities that have reversed and people who avoided many dental expenses and the trauma of fillings and periodontal gum treatments. This simple home care system is a great starting place to improve your mouth health, and if you are prepared to consider some lifestyle and dietary changes, you can expect even more amazing results and long-term financial savings.

My super enjoyable oral health was not inherited from my British family. My father had all his teeth extracted as a preventive measure in the military when he was about thirty years old. I didn't know anything about my mother's oral health until, at forty-five, she was told it was time to have all her teeth extracted and be fitted with full dentures. As a freshman dental student, I knew she had some options, and I was also aware of studies that linked women's loss of their teeth in midlife with an increased risk for dementia. Most of the women in my family were toothless by midlife and had experienced early onset dementia. My mother decided to use my mouth care strategies, and we ended up saving many of her teeth and being able to protect them for the rest of her active and fruitful life. I believe we desperately need to examine this link between oral health and brain health. My mom was always a strong advocate of my protocol and a great example of someone who personally turned her periodontal problems around and retained these teeth for fifty more years, until she died at the ripe age of ninety-five.

WHO SHOULD USE MY SYSTEM?

My Complete Mouth Care System is a daily care mouth program that works alongside xylitol mints and gum to help improve mouth health and protect you from gum disease, cavities, bad breath, sensitivity, and weak teeth. If you already have any of these conditions or if you have been told you need to floss more, I invite you to use all the strategies outlined in this book to improve your mouth's ecology *before* you begin flossing, *before* you have a professional scaling, and *before* you sign up for a course of deep cleanings so that the outcome is far more successful.

Effective home care is essential for anyone who has braces, for anyone with allergies or sinus problems that dry their mouth, for college students who may be living in cramped community conditions where transmission is a risk, for pregnant women who will have acidic saliva throughout pregnancy, for anyone taking medications that dry the mouth, and for anyone who is depressed, stressed, in chemotherapy, or experiencing hormonal fluctuations (especially those associated with aging). Perhaps effective home care will be most important for someone with a family history of any chronic inflammatory conditions (such as diabetes, arthritis, or Lyme disease), for anyone with digestive problems, or for someone who is at risk for cardiovascular disease, stroke, Alzheimer's, or dementia.

HOW OFTEN SHOULD YOU USE THIS SYSTEM?

For the best results, I recommend using all my strategies, but you can experience benefits simply by using xylitol after meals and my suggested rinse system twice daily. At night, our mouth has less protection from saliva, and these drier, more acidic mouth conditions can cause all kinds of dental damage while we sleep. This is why it is important to use an excellent and protective oral care routine every night before going to bed. My system will create ideal conditions for your teeth, so do not eat or drink after using it, with the exception of perhaps having one or two pure xylitol mints if your mouth feels dry. These mints generate a flow of saliva, and this saliva can help mineralize your teeth, especially if you work the saliva around your mouth. During the night, if you wake with a dry mouth and need more mints, they are completely safe to eat.

The second time to use the daily rinse system is generally more flexible, and ideally it should be about twelve hours after the nighttime session, at a time when you will not eat or drink for at least an hour after using it.

PROPER SEQUENCING: YOUR STEPS TO SUSTAINABLE ORAL HEALTH

It is important to follow the rinse protocol in the exact order suggested and to avoid modifying any of the steps except where indicated. Over the past thirty years, I have tried innumerable products to compare them, and it appears to me and thousands of patients that this specific sequencing remains *the* most effective. My previous book, *Kiss Your Dentist Goodbye*, took a close look at how I discovered this sequence of rinsing decades ago, the chemistry of the products involved in each specific step, and why they may create such desirable results and healing. So, if you wish to delve deeper into the science behind the protocol, I encourage you to reference this resource and also my website.

While my strategies may appear simple, and the products are relatively inexpensive, do not be fooled. This is a powerful and effective way to improve your mouth health, and if you give it a try for even a few months, expect to dazzle your dentist with some amazing improvements in the overall health of your mouth at your next visit.

Each of the rinses I suggest targets a number of different mouth problems, and the specific sequencing protects your teeth from any acidity or alcohol that some of the products contain. The system does no harm to healthy bacteria in the mouth, and it promotes dental health benefits quickly, which will make your mouth feel cleaner and healthier.

When beginning my program, I try to ensure you will use the exact products and have clear instructions. I know people who have been so excited to start they purchased incorrect products or they forgot to use the xylitol mints, which are a vital, core component of this system used after every meal, snack, or drink. To find out more about the best way to get the products you need, please visit my website at www.DrEllie.com.

Step 1: Use a Pre-Brushing Rinse with Chlorine Dioxide

The first step of my Complete Mouth Care System is used *before* brushing, and it is a chlorine dioxide rinse. This rinse is useful if you are working to eliminate a deep-seated cavity or periodontal bacteria. This rinse is good at finding its way into tight spaces, and it will travel down the straw-like space to reach cavity bacteria deep inside a tooth. This rinse also targets anaerobic bacteria in infected mouth biofilm and aggressive periodontal pathogens in gum pockets. The oxygen that this rinse generates will help disrupt these problematic bacteria, and I suggest this rinse should be used as the first step of my Complete Mouth Care System, even *before* brushing and definitely before any flossing.

The other parts of this system focus on strengthening teeth, healing cavities, and making teeth smooth so that they will attract less plaque. The toothpaste and final rinse contain a small amount of sodium fluoride, which helps promote absorption of minerals onto the enamel surface for more rapid remineralization of weak areas. As new enamel crystals form and develop, they can actually bridge gaps and span across the enamel surface to heal it and leave it smoother and shinier.

Some dentists have been taught that developing cavities cannot heal and that new enamel merely covers over the decayed area underneath. This is because most dentists in America have used only fluoride, without the benefit of its synergy with xylitol and the usefulness of a chlorine dioxide rinse. Since fluoride does not deal with cavity-causing bacteria, the outcome from using fluoride alone may indeed be bridges of new enamel that cover underlying infection. This is why dentists have experienced situations where they drill through a tiny hole in the hard outer enamel and are shocked to find a soft mush of decay underneath. Do not be disillusioned if your dentist tells you such stories. To ensure that you stop the caries infection completely, you will need to limit your consumption of sugary and acidic drinks and foods and use pure xylitol mints or gum after every meal or snack. Then, this effective home care system, used two or three times per day, will target the anaerobic cavity-causing bacteria of caries, which must be eliminated to allow healing. The other rinses in this system are tools that encourage the cavity to reverse and heal completely.

Many adults end their day with an acidic drink like wine or beer just before brushing their teeth. Teeth are softened by acidity, either from a drink or from acidic saliva in your mouth, and this acidity is hazardous before brushing. Acid-softened teeth are easily abraded, and poorly designed brushes or abrasive toothpaste can make the problem of brushing in an acidic mouth even worse. For this reason, I suggest you begin any toothbrushing routine with a pH-neutral rinse, and this is another attribute of the chlorine dioxide rinse I recommend.

Used alone, chlorine dioxide rinse can be useful if you have gum problems, but when it is used with the complementary parts of my complete system, its benefits appear to be enhanced by the other products. Xylitol and each of the rinses in this system have specific uses, but when they are combined into a targeted strategy, they tackle mouth problems more effectively than any one rinse could do alone. Xylitol is used after meals to nurture healthy oral bacteria, loosen infected plaque, and help develop healthy biofilm. Xylitol has also been shown to work in synergy with dilute sodium fluoride to promote deeper cavity healing.

Step 2: Brush with Sodium Fluoride

The next step after this first chlorine dioxide rinse is to begin brushing, but before you begin, I suggest you put away any expensive, feather-soft toothbrushes and find new medium-strength brushes instead. I also suggest you consider a flossing holiday, especially if you have sensitivity or gum recession. You can gently use some interproximal brushes if necessary but avoid strong antiseptics, peroxide, and baking soda, which will compromise the effectiveness of this system that I recommend.

Xylitol is central to this program, and although it is used during the day, it works in harmony with this system to help keep your gums and teeth bathed in alkaline saliva, mineralizing enamel and nurturing healthy bacteria in your mouth. Xylitol makes infected plaque less sticky, so the rinses and brushing will be very effective.

Sodium fluoride is the fluoride I recommend, and decades of study show it can help mineralize teeth, repair weak enamel, help reverse cavities, protect teeth from enamel erosion, and shorten the normal enamel maturation process for new teeth as they erupt into the mouth. I never recommend stannous fluoride, a cheaper tin-based ingredient that can damage your gums and cause blistering, mouth soreness, and staining. The subject of fluoride has been grossly misunderstood, and if you wish to learn more about why I recommend using topical fluoride but never drinking fluoride, there is a dedicated chapter about the dangers and benefits of fluoride in my book, *Kiss Your Dentist Goodbye*, and further information on my website.

Step 3: Rinse with Acidified Essential Oils

Listerine is a well-known essential oil rinse that was originally formulated in 1879. Listerine tastes strong, which makes everyone think it is an aggressive rinse, but the active ingredients are derived from three essential oils: eucalyptus, menthol, and thymol. A correct combination of essential oils has been shown to penetrate mouth biofilm but not destroy it. Please be aware of the dangers of trying to use other types of essential oils in the mouth as some oils can kill or damage the nerves in teeth, and inappropriate concentrations can be too intense for the skin of your mouth. A well-formulated essential oil rinse will target certain bacteria, especially immature *S. mutans* bacteria. This round, spore-type bacteria is resistant to oxygen and xylitol, so it needs to be addressed in another way to prevent these spores from maturing into sticky plaque, a process which takes about twelve hours.

The potential problem from an acidified essential oil rinse is that alcohol is used to dissolve the oils, and this can cause mouth dryness.

The crisp acidity that is around a pH of 4.2 can also be damaging. This is why acidic mouth rinses should *never* be used unless your tooth enamel has previously been primed with a paste capable of offering adequate protection from the potential for demineralization. This is why it is so important to use the toothpaste that I recommend, which I have confidence will offer this protection. Particularly avoid toothpaste that contains glycerin or the wrong kind or strength of fluoride. For maximum effectiveness, you should use the essential oil rinse vigorously, squeezing and swishing it between your teeth like liquid floss.

When you start using an essential oil rinse for the first time, you may need to adjust your rinsing time, starting out with 5–10 seconds for the first few days or even weeks, and then gradually increasing to 10–20 seconds, until finally 20–40 seconds may be tolerated as your mouth develops adequate biofilm to make this experience comfortable. Never make any alcohol-based rinse the final rinse in your mouth. I suggest this essential-oil step be immediately followed by a protective rinse with dilute sodium fluoride.

Step 4: Rinse with Sodium Fluoride

To protect tooth enamel, I believe it is important to end every meal with a tooth-protective food. In a similar way, I believe it is important to end any mouth care program with a tooth-protective rinse that will ensure there is no mouth-drying alcohol remaining in your mouth. A dilute fluoride rinse is ideal, because it can help stimulate enamel repair and mineralization that will strengthen teeth and improve your tooth color naturally.

A final rinse with these attributes is especially useful if you have damaged or weak teeth, if you have fillings in your teeth, or if you lack natural protection from saliva. I recommend my protocol for anyone with a dry mouth, anyone who develops plaque and calculus, or anyone who has gum problems or feels that their mouth is not as healthy as it used to be. The benefit of using rinses is that they enter all the small crevices and grooves in your teeth, even under and around braces, crowns, or bridgework, to strengthen places that are often the most inaccessible to a toothbrush and often the places where cavities begin.

A few drops of mouth rinse will work just as well as a large mouthful. Most mouth rinse manufacturers encourage you to use as much as possible, but I have found no science to connect the mouth benefits with the volume of rinse used. With any mouth rinse, feel free to be economical with your rinse volume. Maximize the benefits of your final protective rinse by not eating or drinking for at least an hour after you finish the routine, and spit out the last rinse.

Most categories of oral care products appear to vary their formulations regularly. This is why it is difficult to write about specific products by name. In my book, *Kiss Your Dentist Goodbye*, I discuss specific products and why they were selected, but please check my website for the latest details and updated product information.

Step 5: Clean Your Toothbrush

Your toothbrush should be stored properly between uses. I recommend placing it in a kitchen window or any clean location far away from a bathroom toilet, which can spread toilet bacteria up to 10 feet in the air, even with the lid down. Before storing your toothbrush, it is important to clean it, and an essential oil rinse like Listerine can help remove bacteria from your brush. You can pour a few drops of this rinse on your brush, or dip and swish your brush in a small capful of the liquid. Then, rinse the brush in water before storing it head-up so the bristles can dry for twenty-four hours between uses.

AN OUNCE OF PREVENTION

Before you have tooth problems or think you have a cavity, I urge you to try my system of care and see if you can improve your mouth health. Once you have dental disease and visible problems or pain, you will already be on a downward spiral. The longer you wait to reverse direction, the more difficult your turnaround will become. Remember, many things can sabotage your efforts, so this is not the time to try to improve on product recommendations or add things that you think could possibly be helpful. Too many patients have tried using harsh chemicals and been unsuccessful, and baking soda, peroxide, and even tea tree oil can be damaging to healthy bacteria or strip biofilm proteins that are the necessary foundation for mouth health.

Some recent testing indicates that extended sessions of oil pulling with coconut oil can kill the good as well as the bad bacteria. Stronger fluoride pastes or gels may also be damaging, and I suggest you avoid bleach, iodine, or antibiotics, which can derail your progress.

At the heart of your mouth's recovery should be the understanding of why you had problems in the past. Think about a day in the life of your teeth, and consider everything you subject them to on a daily basis—from the moment you wake up until you go to bed. One time I was exploring why a young lady had spent thousands of dollars on root canals and crowns because of agonizing tooth sensitivity. In the first five minutes of our conversation, she explained how every day she prepared lemon wedges as a refreshing snack. This daily habit, sucking acidic lemons, had caused a devastating and expensive demineralization problem for her lower front teeth.

Another time, I discovered corrosive phytates stripping the enamel of someone who regularly snacked on raw kale and spinach. I have also alerted smoothie-sipping, coffee-clutching, iced-tea loving, and lemonade-drinking clients about these often healthy but tooth-dangerous habits. In the same way, sugary candies and mints, vitamin C lozenges, and cough syrup can be dental hazards.

My Complete Mouth Care System is a great tool to defend your teeth and gums from damage and dental infections, but I encourage you to consider the various habits you have and determine which ones may be contributing to poor oral health. Remember that the outcome for teeth is the balance of a simple equation between the total damage your teeth endure each day versus the total amount of mineralization and repair they experience each day. There is no magic bullet for mouth health, and the best guidance is to keep potentially damaging foods and drinks—especially sodas, juices, candies, or lemon wedges—to mealtimes and always end meals and snacks with a tooth-protective food or some pure xylitol gum or mints.

FLOSSING

Many people blame their dental problems on excuses that include a lack of fluoride, no access to dentistry, inadequate dental insurance, or insufficient flossing. We have discussed in detail that dental problems do not begin because of a lack of drinking fluoride, and they cannot be stopped by a dentist or by flossing. Dental problems always begin with some type of acidic damage that provides the environment for aggressive, acid-loving bacteria. These bacteria may have transferred from people in your family or from friends around you, but they needed to be sustained in your mouth by sugar or carbohydrates in your diet or drinks. The problem is that, once these harmful bacteria gain control, only targeted strategies like mine can change your mouth situation and truly restore it to health.

I am not against flossing per se, and if someone wants to floss in a healthy mouth, and does so carefully, this may be harmless. As we discussed in chapter 6, I believe flossing in an infected mouth can be a health problem, and unnecessary flossing or overflossing can easily make teeth sensitive, cause gums to recede, and put people at risk for pushing plaque bacteria into the blood, with the potential to contribute to plaque in arteries or worse. If you have poor mouth health and have been told to floss, I suggest you explore my method of mouth care first, as it may be an easier, more effective, and less risky route to cleaner gums and healthier teeth. If you have a healthy mouth and like to floss, I believe the best time to floss is when you have toothpaste on your teeth, so a small amount of paste will be pulled and pushed between the interproximal areas between teeth. This way of using floss to move toothpaste could also be useful if you are trying to heal interproximal cavities between your teeth, since it will ensure the toothpaste has access to help mineralize these areas on your teeth.

WORKING WITH NEW PATIENTS

Hundreds of success stories from patients using my Complete Mouth Care System have illustrated how gum disease and cavities can reverse and heal under correct conditions. These patients have witnessed their teeth becoming brighter and healthier with every passing year, even into their seventies and eighties! This is why I encourage everyone to try the system, but there is a caveat: The speed and completeness of mouth improvements are closely associated with general body health, which is why I encourage a full protocol that factors in diet, exercise, stress management, smart sun exposure for Vitamin D production, supplements as necessary, a healthy amount of sleep, and good daily nutrition.

When I work with a new patient, my first concern—before I detail the status of their teeth—is to ask some questions about their general health. In my experience, teeth and gums do not automatically deteriorate with age if we remain aware of the factors that are risks to mouth health and the importance of nutrition and digestive health on saliva quality. Without adequate care and effective strategies, dental diseases can easily progress and cause ongoing damage to your teeth year after year.

—

In the 1990s, I was giving public seminars to teach truths about oral health before we had the convenience of websites and blogs. I rented a conference room and tried to entertain my audience with the science of gum disease and cavities, showing them how to measure mouth pH, and what happens to an egg when it is immersed in soda for a few hours. An acquaintance of mine, a lady in her fifties, was an attendee at one of these events. She was smart, highly educated, and definitely understood the science of this subject. At the end of the session I gave guests a complimentary kit containing xylitol mints and all the oral care products I suggested for their home care. Hundreds of people came to these events, and their successes ignited a fan base that has continued to grow over the years, with incredible stories of healing and sustained oral health.

This one friend, however, was not confident to try the products without first asking advice from her dentist. She took the products to his office, and he determined it was rubbish. He suggested other things, and she followed his advice, not mine. With hectic lives, we did not see each other for the next fifteen years, and I was stunned, saddened, and shocked when we accidentally bumped into each other in a store and she smiled at me. I could not believe the damage that had happened to her mouth—lost teeth, crowns, gum disease, and probably more.

During those fifteen years, I believe she could have enjoyed oral health and perhaps avoided the need for any dental treatments, but instead she obviously experienced the dental drama that can easily occur in postmenopausal years, when a drier mouth and mouth acidity are caused by hormone fluctuations. There is a predictable pattern of disease that often occurs in these years as teeth become sensitive, fillings need replacement, and fractures or erosion lead to root canals and crowns. A dental crown stresses opposing teeth, which can cause more damage and can lead to more extractions, implants, and ongoing dental damage.

Ultimately, in acidic and dry mouth conditions, the gums will show signs of damage, and after all these dental woes, many people discover their teeth loosen, and they will need more frequent cleanings, gum surgery, and perhaps eventually dentures. No amount of flossing and brushing addresses the underlying acidity and dry mouth problems adequately.

How I wish my friend had used my system. I am confident she could have avoided most or all of this damage. The use of correct products can balance the mouth ecology and put an end to progressive, destructive disease, which sadly can destroy many of the teeth in the mouths of patients at retirement age. I respect her wanting professional endorsement, but I am saddened that she had to endure so much damage to her mouth health. For my friend, the damage has been done, but I encourage you to start the Complete Mouth Care System as soon as possible and try to avoid this awful cycle before it starts.

TESTIMONIALS

Over my career, I have received thousands of testimonials from patients who were told they needed cavities filled or expensive gum therapies, but after using my Complete Mouth Care System, they returned to their dentist to discover that their problems had vanished. Unless treatment is an emergency, and before setting a date for fillings, I suggest you follow my protocol for a few months to improve your mouth's ecology and encourage mitigation of damage.

Dr. Christine Landes, DMD, is a pediatric dentist who decided to implement a novel preventive program in her Newton Dentistry office in Newton, Pennsylvania some years ago, documenting the number of fillings her office could *prevent* in their young patients' mouths. In one year, their records showed they saved children from a total of 1,600 fillings by recommending xylitol and good home care methods. They said it had reduced the amount of work in their office, they found the results exciting, and everyone slept well at night knowing it was the right thing to do. This office continues to help children remain cavity-free, and in 2017, they told me that they had avoided $70,000 worth of fillings. This office is centered on health education and is a huge proponent of xylitol.

NEW DIRECTIONS

There seems to be enormous interest in finding a pathway to oral wellness. This makes me hopeful that times are changing and that finally people understand the value of true mouth health and are less excited about fancy photo sessions and fake, overly white smiles. On the other hand, this brings us back to one of our first questions: How do you judge mouth health?

To achieve success, we must address diet and oral bacteria—good and bad. We must understand that bacteria are transmissible and will pass in droplets of saliva as friends and families kiss, talk, or share food with one other. If we want healthy teeth, we will not find the answer in a tube of toothpaste or a roll of floss. Our goal must be to promote the conditions that nurture a healthy mouth ecology so that our own mouth health will, in fact, defend us from dental problems.

Sensitive teeth, bad breath, cavities, and gum disease are all symptoms of a problem—a mouth ecosystem that is unhealthy and out of balance. If you want a healthier mouth, I'd suggest that you try my protocol and work to improve your general health through diet and improved habits. As your oral, nasal, sinus, and digestive health improves, you will usually find that any sensitivity, bad breath, and cavities, will disappear—hopefully forever.

Thank you for your interest in reading this book, which I hope will bring you encouragement and hope.

Wishing you good health and happiness,
Ellie Phillips, DDS

References

CHAPTER 1

1. W.V. Giannobil, T.M. Braun, A.K. Capli, L. Doucette-Stamm, G.W. Duff, K.S. Kornman. "Patient Stratification for Preventive Care in Dentistry." *Journal of Dental Research.* 2013 August; 92(8): 694-701.

CHAPTER 2

1. N.C. Foley, R.H. Affoo, W.L. Siqueira, R.E. Martin. "A Systematic Review Examining the Oral Health Status of Persons with Dementia." *Journal of Clinical and Translational Research.* 2017 October; 2(4): 330-342.

2. J. Ahn. "Certain Oral Bacteria Associated with Increased Pancreatic Cancer Risk." Presented at the American Association for Cancer Research (AACR) Annual Meeting. 2016 April.

3. Peer Reviewed: Bale-Doneen study. Discussion, "How Bacteria in Your Mouth Can Harm Your Heart." Healthy Hearts, Healthy Practices.

4. B.F. Bale, A.L. Doneen, D.J. Vigerust. "High-risk Periodontal Pathogens Contribute to the Pathogenesis of Artherosclerosis." *Postgraduate Medical Journal.* 2016 November.

5. X. Li, K.M. Koltveit, L. Tronstad, I. Olsen. "Systemic Diseases Caused by Oral Infection." *Clinical Microbiology Reviews.* 2000 October; 13(4):547-558.

6. R. Saini, S. Saini, S.R. Saini. "Periodontitis: A Risk for Delivery of Premature Labor and Low-Birth-Weight Infants." *Journal of Natural Science, Biology and Medicine.* 2010 July-December; 1(1): 40-42.

7. S.G. Fitzpatrick, J. Katz. "The association between Periodontal Disease and Cancer: a Review of the Literature." *Journal of Dentistry.* 2010 February; 38(2):83-95.

8. P.M. Preshaw, A.L. Alba, D. Herrera, S. Jepsen, A. Konstantinidis, K. Makrilakis, R. Taylor. "Periodontitis and Diabetes: A Two-Way Relationship." *Diabetologia.* 2012 January; 55(1): 21-31.

9. G.R. Persson. "Rheumatoid Arthritis and Periodontitis - Inflammatory

and Infectious Connections. Review of the Literature." *Journal of Oral Microbiology.* 2012; 4.

10. B. F. Teixeira, M.T. Saito, F.C. Matheur, R.D. Prediger, E.S. Yamada, C.S.F. Maia, R.R. Lima. "Periodontitis and Alzheimer's Disease: A Possible Comorbidity between Oral Chronic Inflammatory Condition and Neuroinflammation." *Frontiers in Aging Neuroscience.* 2017; 9:327.

11. G.D. Ehrlich, F.Z. Hu, N. Sotereanos, J. Sewicke, J. Parvizi, P.L. Nara, C.R. Arciola. "What Role Do Periodontal Pathogens Play in Osteoarthritis and Periprosthetic Joint Infections of the Knee?" *Journal of Applied Biomaterials.* 2014 June; 12(1).

12. S. Paju, J. Oittinen, H. Haapala, S. Asikainen, J. Paavonen, P.J. Pussinen. "*Porphyromonas gingivalis* may Interfere with Conception in Women." *Journal of Oral Microbiology.* 2017 June; 9(1).

13. J. Katz, N. Chegini, K.T. Shiverick, R.J. Lamont. "Localization of *P. gingivalis* in Preterm Delivery Placenta." *Journal of Dental Research.* 2009 June; 88(6): 575-8.

14. J.A. Haworth, H.F. Jenkinson, H.J. Petersen, C.R. Back, J.L. Brittan, S.W. Kerrigan, A.H. Nobbs. "Concerted Functions of *S. gordonii* Surface Proteins PadA and Hsa mediater Activation of Human Platelets and Interactions with Extracellular Matrix." *Cellular Microbiology.* 2017 January: 19(1).

15. J. Abranches, J.H. Miller, A.R. Martinez, P.J. Simpson-Haldaris, R.A. Bume, J.A. Lemos. "The Collagen-Binding Protein Cnm is Required for *Streptococcus mutans* Adherence to and Intracellular Invasion of Human Coronary Artery Endothelial Cells." *Infectious Immunity.* 2011 June; 79 (6): 2277-84.

16. M.K. Jeffcoat, N.C. Geurs, M.S. Reddy, S.P. Cliver, R.L. Goldenberg, J.C. Hauth. "Periodontal Infection and Preterm Birth." *Journal of the American Dental Association.* 2001; 132(7): 875-880.

17. R.L. Goldenberg, J.F. Culhane, J.D. Iams, R. Romero. "Epidemiology and Causes Of Preterm Birth." *Lancet.* 2008 January 5; 371(9606): 75-84.

18. N.J. Lopez, P.C. Smith, J. Gutierrez. "Higher Risk of Preterm Birth and Low Birth Weight in Women with Periodontal Disease." *Journal of Dental Research.* 2002; 81(1): 58-63.

19. B.S. Michalowicz, J.S. Hodges, A.J. DiAngelis, V.R. Lupo, M.J. Novak, J.E. Ferguson, W. Buchanan, J. Bofill, P.N. Papapanou, D.A. Mitchell, S. Matseoane, P.A. Tschida, "Treatment of Periodontal Disease and the Risk of Preterm Birth." *The New England Journal of Medicine.* 2006; 355: 1885-1894.

20. K.A. Boggess, B.L. Edelstein. "Oral Health in Women During Preconception and Pregnancy: Implications for Birth Outcomes and Infant Oral Health." *Maternal Child Health Journal.* 2006 September; 10 (supplement 1): 169-174.

21. K. Aagaard, J. Ma, K.M. Anthony, R. Ganu, J. Petrosiono, J. Versalovic. "The placenta harbors a unique microbiome." *Science Translational Medicine.* 2014 May 21; 6(237): 237.

CHAPTER 3

1. M.R. Frazelle, C.L. Munro. "Toothbrush Contamination: A Review of the Literature." *Nursing Research and Practice.* 2012; 2012: 420-630.

2. A. Mehta, P.S. Sequeira, G. Bhat. "Bacterial Contamination and Decontamination of Toothbrushes After Use." *New York State Dental Journal.* 2007 April; 73(3): 20-2.

3. E. S. Frenkel and K. Ribbeck. "Salivary Mucins Protect Surfaces From Colonization by Cariogenic Bacteria." *Applied and Environmental Microbiology.* 2015; 81(1): 332-338.

CHAPTER 4

1. J.E.Kim, M.G. Ferruzzi, W.W. Campbell. "Egg Consumption Increases Vitamin E Absorption from Co-Consumed Raw Mixed Vegetables in Healthy Young Men." *The Journal of Nutrition.* 2016; 146: 2199-2205.

2. M. Kushiyama, Y. Shimazaki, M. Murakami, Y. Yamashita. "Relationship Between Intake of Green Tea and Periodontal Disease." *Journal of Periodontology.* 2009 March; 80(3): 372-377.

3. B. Kargul, M. Ozcan, S. Peker, T. Nakamoto, W.B. Simmons, A.U. Falster. "Evaluation of Human Enamel Surfaces Treated with Theobromine: A Pilot Study." *Oral Health & Preventive Dentistry.* 2012; 10(3): 275-82.

4. I. Gedalia, D. Ionat-Bendat, S. Ben-Mosheh, L. Shapira. "Tooth Enamel Softening with a Cola Type Drink and Rehardening With Hard Cheese or Stimulated Saliva." *Journal of Oral Rehabilitation.* 1991; 18: 501-506.

5. M.E. Thompson quoted in M. Edgar, "Diet, Functional Foods, and Oral Health," in *Functional Foods, Ageing, and Degenerative Disease.* eds. C. Remacle and B. Reusen (London: Woodhead Publishing Limited, 2004).

CHAPTER 5

1. A. Consolaro, L.A. Francischone, R.B. Consolaro. "Tooth Whitening Products in Toothpastes and Mouthwashes." *Orthodontic Insight. Journal of Orthodontics.* 2011 March-April; 16(2): 28-35.

2. C.E. Berchier, D.E. Slot, S. Haps, G.A. Van der Weijden. "The Efficacy of Dental Floss In Addition to a Toothbrush On Plaque and Parameters of Gingival Inflammation: A Systematic Review." *International Journal of Dental Hygiene.* 2008; 6: 265-279.

3. C.S. Louis. "Feeling Guilty About Not Flossing? Maybe there's no Need." *New York Times* Associated Press News Article. August 2, 2016.

CHAPTER 6

1. P.T. Mattila, M.J. Svanberg, M.L. Knuuttila. "Increased Bone Volume and Bone Mineral Content in Xylitol-fed Aged Rats." *Gererontology.* 2001 November-December; 47(6): 300-5.

2. A. Azarpazhooh, H.P. Lawrence, P.S. Shah. "Xylitol for Preventing Acute Otitis Media in Children up to 12 years of Age." *Cochrane Database, Systematic Review.* 2016 August.

3. P.A. Nayak, U.A. Nayak, V. Khandelwal. "The Effect of Xylitol on Dental Caries and Oral Flora." *Clinical, Cosmetic and Investigational Dentistry.* 2014; 6: 89-94.

4. Y. Nakai, C. Shinga-Ishihara, M. Kaji, K. Mariya, K. Murakami-Yamanaka, M. Takimura. "Xylitol Gum and Maternal Transmission of Mutans Streptococci." *Journal of Dental Research.* 2010 January; 89(1): 56-60.

5. K.K. Makinen, C.A. Bennett, P.P. Hujoel, P.J. Isokangas, K.P. Isotupa, H.R. Pape Jr., P.L. Makinen. "Xylitol Chewing Gums and Caries Rates: a 40-month Cohort Study." *Journal of Dental Research.* 1995 December; 74 (12): 1904-13.

6. T. Tapiainen, T. Kontiokari, L. Sammalkivi, I. Ikaheimo, M. Koskela, M. Uhari. "Effect of Xylitol on Growth of *Streptococcus pneumoniae* in the Presence of Fructose and Sorbitol." *Antimicobial Agents and Chemotherapy.* 2001 January; 45(1): 166-169.

7. A. Rivière, M. Selak, D. Lantin, F. Leroy, L.D. Vuyst. "Bifidobacteria and Butyrate-Producing Colon Bacteria: Importance and Strategies for their stimulation in the Human Gut." *Frontiers in Microbiology.* 2016; 7: 979.

8. P. Milgrom, K. Ly, M.C. Roberts, M. Rothen, G. Muller, D.K. Yamaguchi. "Mutans Streptococci Dose Response to Xylitol Chewing Gum." *Journal of Dental Research.* 2006 February; 85(2): 177-181.

9. P. Milgrom, K.A. Ly, O.K. Tut, L. Manci, M.C. Roberts, K. Briand, M.J. Gancio. "Xylitol Pediatric Topical Oral Syrup to Prevent Dental Caries: A Double Blind, Randomized Clinical Trial of Efficacy." *Archives of Pediatric Adolescent Medicine.* 2009 July; 163(7): 601-607.

10. V.I. Haraszthy, J.J. Zambon, P.K. Sreenivasan, M.M. Zambon, D. Gerber, R. Rego, C. Parker. "Identification of Oral Bacterial Species Associated with Halitosis." *Journal of the American Dental Association.* 2007 August; 138(8): 1113-20.

11. T. Takeshita, N Suzuki, Y Nakano, Y. Shimazaki, M. Yoneda, T. Hirofuji, Y. Yamashita. "Relationship between Oral Malodor and the Global Composition of Indigenous Bacterial Populations in Saliva." *Applied and Environmental Microbiology.* 2010 May; 76(9): 2806-2814.

CHAPTER 7

1. B. Hesselmar, F. Sjoberg, R. Saalman, N. Aberg, I. Adlerberth, A.E. Wold. "Pacifier Cleaning Practices and Risk of Allergy Development." *Pediatrics.* 2013 May.

2. W.H. Bowen, R.A. Lawrence. "Comparison of the Cariogenicity of Cola, Honey, Cow Milk, Human Milk, and Sucrose." *Pediatrics.* 2005 October; 116(4): 921-6.

3. R. Widome. "What can Oral Public Health Learn From Finland?" *American Journal of Public Health.* 2004 November; 94(11).

4. I. Arpalahti, T. Mimmi, P. Kaisu. "Comparing Health Promotion Programs in Public Dental Service of Vantaa, Finland: A Clinical Trial in 6–36-Month-Old Children." *International Journal of Dentistry.* 2013; 2013: 757-938.

CHAPTER 8

1. F. Nejatidanesh, Z. Khoosravi, H. Goroohi, H. Badrian, O. Savabi. "Risk of Contamination of Different Areas of Dentist's Face During Dental Practices." *International Journal of Preventive Medicine.* 2013 May; 4(5): 611-615.

2. J. Petersson. "Nitrates, Nitrite and Nitric Oxide in Gastric Mucosal Defense." *Uppsala University, Faculty of Medicine.* 2008.

3. E.B. Claus, L. Calvocoressi, M.L. Bondy, J.M. Schildkraut, J.L. Wiemeis, M. Wrensch. "Dental X-rays and Risk of Meningioma." *Cancer.* 2012 September; 118(18): 4530-7.

4. H.J. Keene and I.L. Shklair. "Relationship of *Streptococcus mutans* Carrier Status to the Development of Carious Lesions in Initially Caries Free Recruits." *Journal of Dental Research.* 1974; 53: 1295.

COLLECTIVE

1. J.A. Haworth, H.F. Jenkinson, H.J. Petersen, C.R. Back, J.L. Brittan, S.W. Kerrigan, A.H. Nobbs. "Concerted functions of *Streptococcus gordonii* surface proteins PadA and Hsa mediate activation of human platelets and interactions with extracellular matrix." *The National Center for Biotechnology Information* 2017 January; https://www.ncbi.nlm.nih.gov/pubmed/27616700.

Index

conditions related with dental and gum disease, 20–27

Dr. Ron Phillips's on, 27–28

and health seekers, 28–29

and nurturing healthy mouth bacteria, 24–25

overview, 17–18

and periodontal pathogens, 20–22, 24

preterm births, 26–27

transmission of dental disease, 18–19, 35–37

See also bodily health

health benefits

of food pairing, 61–62

healthy biofilm, 49

of xylitol, 114–16, 118–19

heart disease and heart attacks, 17, 24, 25–26, 41. *See also* cardiovascular health

high blood pressure, and gum disease, 23

hip replacements, 25

history of dentistry

American Dental Association (ADA), 2

cleanings, 11–14

cosmetic dentistry, 3–4

dental marketing, 5–6

dental-restoration era, 2–3

extractions in order to solve medical problems, 1

focus on removing bad bacteria, 4–5

maintenance of fillings, 8–9

new techniques and equipment, 14–15

periodontal treatment, 9–10

silver amalgam fillings, 1–2

sustainable oral health, 15–16

treatment ladder, 7–8

homemade toothpastes, 53, 63, 163–64

hormones/hormonal changes, 39, 51, 74, 98, 104, 133, 166, 175–76

hot and cold, teeth sensitivity, 45, 47

Hubbard, Elbert, 1

Human Microbiome Project, 33, 72

hydrogen peroxide. *See* peroxide

hygiene model of dental practice, 159–60

I

immune system

and biofilm health, 48

and blood flow to gums, 106

boosting before a dental visit, 152

dental cleanings and a compromised, 25

and digestive health, 52, 53, 59–60

foods boosting, 67, 72, 124

and gingivitis, 39–40

and nutrition, 59–60

and periodontal pathogens, 21, 27, 41

incomplete lip closure, 81

infants, xylitol for, 117. *See also* babies

infected toothbrushes, 112

infection(s)

around dental implants, 10

from bacteria in dental water lines, 14

baking soda/peroxide poultice for gum, 99

dentistry approach to masking underlying, 2, 3

digestive health and fighting, 74

gum. *See* periodontal disease

lung, 47–48

middle-ear, 23, 47–48, 115

periodontal pathogens causing, 41

remaining after dental treatments, 8

sinus, 23

on toothbrushes, 35–37

and tooth sensitivity, 45

infertility-treatment failure, and gum disease, 23

inflammation

and digestive health, 53

and heart disease, 24

from periodontal pathogens, 41

systemic, xvii, xx

See also body inflammation; periodontal disease

Inspektor Research Systems light technology, 154

insurance companies/industry, 78–79, 153–54, 159

interdental brushes, 108

International Dental Journal, 95

.

About the Author

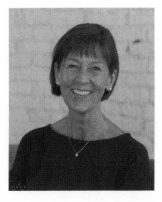 Dr. Ellie discovered early in her dental career that she could help people reverse cavities and gum disease. Her first educational program launched in 1975 to teach pregnant women how to improve their dental health and care for their children's teeth. For four decades, she has worked to unravel dental science and help patients understand why cavities and gum disease happen and what can prevent these problems.

Dr. Ellie believes oral health is a choice and that teeth are too valuable to accept the myth that cavities and gum disease are genetic or simply inevitable. She believes anyone can improve their oral health and that most dental problems are avoidable and reversible. She promotes home care strategies and has shared her knowledge as a consultant, speaker, and author of numerous articles and books over many decades.

Dr. Ellie's dental experiences in England, Switzerland, and the United States have given her a broad view of dentistry and an interest in many specialties and patients of all ages. She has a background in oral surgery, community dentistry, general practice, geriatric dental care, and cosmetic dentistry. She is a pediatric specialist and was the pediatric clinic director and a member of the dental faculty at the University of Rochester. During her professional career, she was a member of the American Dental Association, the American Academy of Pediatric Dentistry, and an Honorary Member of the Eastman Institute for Oral Health, U.K. Her lifelong interest in health and wellness led her to become a founding member of the American Academy for Oral Systemic Health, and in

2005, she founded a company that creates and promotes xylitol supplements for oral health.

Dr. Ellie lives in Austin, Texas and is deeply involved in the lives of
her five children and grandchildren, but she remains dedicated to her
mission: to help as many people as possible achieve sustainable oral health
and enjoy the whole-body benefits associated with a healthier mouth.

Made in the USA
Las Vegas, NV
17 May 2024

90024446R00134